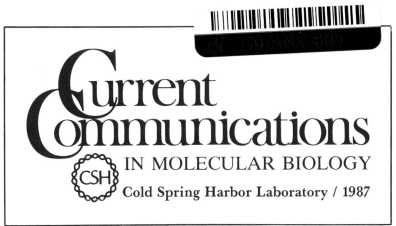

Current Communications

IN MOLECULAR BIOLOGY

(CSH) Cold Spring Harbor Laboratory / 1987

Angiogenesis

Mechanisms and Pathobiology

Edited by

Daniel B. Rifkin

New York University Medical Center

Michael Klagsbrun

Harvard University Medical School

Titles in
Current Communications in Molecular Biology
PLANT INFECTIOUS AGENTS
ENHANCERS AND EUKARYOTIC GENE EXPRESSION
PROTEIN TRANSPORT AND SECRETION
IMMUNE RECOGNITION OF PROTEIN ANTIGENS
EUKARYOTIC TRANSCRIPTION
PLANT CELL/CELL INTERACTIONS
TRANSLATIONAL CONTROL
COMPUTER GRAPHICS AND MOLECULAR MODELING
MICROBIAL ENERGY TRANSDUCTION
MECHANISMS OF YEAST RECOMBINATION
DNA PROBES
GENE TRANSFER VECTORS FOR MAMMALIAN CELLS
ANGIOGENESIS Mechanisms and Pathobiology

ANGIOGENESIS Mechanisms and Pathobiology
© 1987 by Cold Spring Harbor Laboratory
All rights reserved
International Standard Book Number 0-87969-300-2
Book design by Emily Harste
Printed in the United States of America

Cover: Growth of blood vessels in the rat cornea toward an implant of an ELVAX (ethylene-vinyl acetate copolymer) pellet containing about 50 ng of chondrosarcoma tumor-derived endothelial cell growth factor. (Photo courtesy of M. Klagsbrun.)

All Cold Spring Harbor Laboratory publications may be ordered directly from Cold Spring Harbor Laboratory, Box 100, Cold Spring Harbor, New York 11724. (Phone: Continental U.S. except New York State 1-800-843-4388. All other locations [516]367-8425.)

Conference Participants

Robert Auerbach, Dept. of Zoology, University of Wisconsin, Madison
Michael J. Banda, Laboratory of Radiobiology, University of California, San Francisco
Denis Barritault, Université Paris, France
Peter Böhlen, Biochemisches Institut, Universität Zurich, Switzerland
John Castellot, Dept. of Pathology, Harvard University Medical School, Boston, Massachusetts
Yves Courtois, INSERM, Paris, France
Patricia A. D'Amore, Laboratory of Surgical Research, The Children's Hospital, Boston, Massachusetts
Jeffrey M. Davidson, Dept. of Pathology, Vanderbilt University School of Medicine, Nashville, Tennessee
Rik Derynck, Genentech, Inc., South San Francisco, California
Paul E. DiCorleto, Cleveland Clinic Research Institute, Ohio
John C. Fiddis, California Biotechnology Inc., Mountain View, California
Judah Folkman, Dept. of Surgical Research, Harvard University Medical School, Boston, Massachusetts
Michael Fox, Amgen, Thousand Oaks, California
Raj Ghai, Ciba-Geigy Corporation, Summit, New Jersey
Bert M. Glaser, Johns Hopkins Hospital, Baltimore, Maryland
Leslie Gold, Oncogene Science, Inc., Mineola, New York
Christian Haudenschild, Boston University School of Medicine, Massachusetts
Hanne M. Jensen, Dept. of Pathology, University of California, Davis
Michael Klagsbrun, Harvard University Medical School, Boston, Massachusetts
David R. Knighton, University of Minnesota Hospital, Minneapolis
Shant Kumar, Christie Hospital and Holt Radium Institute, Manchester, England
Thomas Maciag, Biotechnology Research Center, Rockville, Maryland
David Moscatelli, Dept. of Cell Biology, New York University Medical Center, New York
Anthony Neri, Hoffmann-La Roche Inc., Nutley, New Jersey
Maurice Petitou, Institut Choay, Paris, France
Daniel B. Rifkin, Dept. of Cell Biology, New York University Medical Center, New York
Werner Risau, Max-Planck Institut für Entwicklungsbiologie, Tubingen, Federal Republic of Germany
Anita B. Roberts, National Cancer Institute, Bethesda, Maryland
Robert D. Rosenberg, Massachusetts Institute of Technology, Cambridge
Milton M. Sholley, Dept. of Anatomy, Virginia Commonwealth University, Richmond

Andreas Sommer, Synergen, Inc., Boulder, Colorado

Kenneth A. Thomas, Dept. of Biochemistry and Molecular Biology, Merck Sharp & Dohme Research Laboratories, Rahway, New Jersey

Mary Treuhaft, Schering Corporation, Bloomfield, New Jersey

Israel Vlodavsky, Dept. of Radiation and Clinical Oncology, Hadassah University Hospital, Jerusalem, Israel

John W. Wilks, Cancer and Viral Diseases Research, The Upjohn Company, Kalamazoo, Michigan

Preface

The process of angiogenesis has always been attractive as an experimental system, since the formation of capillary sprouts involves a single responsive cell type and can be initiated by a number of controlled procedures. There has been intense interest in understanding the mechanisms controlling angiogenesis because of the relevance of neovascularization to normal physiology as well as to disease states such as cancer and arthritis.

Early experiments studying neovascularization were focused on demonstrating the existence of molecules responsible for both the initiation and the inhibition of blood vessel growth, as well as the development of suitable assay systems such as the rabbit cornea, the chick chorioallantoic membrane, and the hamster cheek pouch. In the past 5 years, in vitro assays were developed for putative angiogenesis factors as efforts were mounted to isolate the controlling molecules for this process. These approaches have recently resulted in the isolation of several proteins capable of inducing angiogenesis at low doses in vivo. Attention now has shifted to an analysis of the molecular and cell biology of these molecules in normal and pathological states.

It thus seemed appropriate at this time to bring together individuals interested in a wide spectrum of areas concerned with angiogenesis, and a conference on angiogenesis was held at the Banbury Center of Cold Spring Harbor Laboratory in November 1986. The extended abstracts of the presentations made at the meeting are summarized in this volume and cover aspects of the molecular biology, cell biology, pathophysiology, and therapeutic use of angiogenic factors and inhibitors.

The convivial surroundings of the Banbury Center fostered a remarkable atmosphere for intellectual exchange. Most of the credit for this must go to Steve Prentis and Bea Toliver of the Banbury Center for handling the organizational efforts; to Katya Davey and her staff at the Robertson House for their hospitality; and to Jim Watson for his encouragement and support for the initial idea of holding such a meeting at Banbury. Additional thanks are due to Nancy Ford, Chris Nolan, and Mary Cozza for their outstanding help in editing and publishing this volume.

D.B.R.
M.K.

The meeting on Angiogenesis was funded entirely by proceeds from the Laboratory's Corporate Sponsor Program, whose members provide core support for Cold Spring Harbor and Banbury meetings:

Abbott Laboratories
American Cyanamid Company
Amersham International plc
Becton Dickinson and Company
Cetus Corporation
Ciba-Geigy Corporation
CPC International Inc.
E.I. du Pont de Nemours & Company
Eli Lilly and Company
Genentech, Inc.
Genetics Institute
Hoffmann-La Roche Inc.
Monsanto Company
Pall Corporation
Pfizer Inc.
Schering-Plough Corporation
Smith Kline & French Laboratories
Tambrands Inc.
The Upjohn Company
Wyeth Laboratories

Contents

Conference Participants, iii
Preface, v

Introduction   1
M. Klagsbrun

Structure and Activities of Acidic Fibroblast Growth
Factor   9
K. Thomas, G. Gimenez-Gallego, J. DiSalvo,
D. Linemeyer, L. Kelly, J. Menke, T. Mellin, and
R. Busch

Multiple Forms of Hepatoma-derived Basic Fibroblast
Growth Factor: Cleavages by Tumor Cell Acid
Proteinases   13
M. Klagsburn

Endothelial Cell Growth Factor   18
T. Maciag

Genes for the Angiogenic Growth Factors, Basic and
Acidic Fibroblast Growth Factors   24
J.C. Fiddes, J.L. Whang, A. Mergia, A. Tumolo, and
J.A. Abraham

Primary Structure of a Human Basic Fibroblast Growth
Factor Derived from Protein and cDNA Sequencing   32
A. Sommer, M.T. Brewer, R.C. Thompson, D. Moscatelli,
M. Presta, and D.B. Rifkin

Modulation of Eye-derived Growth Factor Activity and
Fixation in the Eye   37
Y. Courtois

A Heparin Hexasaccharide Fragment Able to Bind to
Anionic Endothelial Cell Growth Factor: Preparation and
Structure   43
J.C. Lormeau, M. Petitou, J. Choay, and B. Perly

Presence of Basic Fibroblast Growth Factor in a Variety
of Cells and Its Binding to Cells 47
D. Moscatelli, M. Presta, J. Joseph-Silverstein,
and D.B. Rifkin

Eye-derived Fibroblast Growth Factors: Receptors and
Early Event Studies 52
M. Moenner, J. Badet, B. Chevallier, M. Tardieu,
J. Courty, and D. Barritault

Heparin-binding Endothelial Cell Growth Factors Are
Sequestered by the Extracellular Matrix 58
I. Vlodavsky, J. Folkman, and M. Klagsbrun

Production of Platelet-derived Growth Factor-like Protein
by Endothelial Cells 65
P.E. DiCorleto, P.L. Fox, and G.M. Chisolm

Transforming Growth Factor-β: Stimulator or Inhibitor
of Angiogenesis? 69
A.B. Roberts and M.B. Sporn

Transforming Growth Factor-α Induces Angiogenesis 72
R. Derynck, M.E. Winkler, and A.B. Schreiber

Nonpeptide Angiogenesis Factors 78
C.C. Haudenschild and M.I. Klibaner

Differentiation-dependent Stimulation of Angiogenesis by
3T3-Adipocytes 85
J.J. Castellot, Jr. and B.M. Spiegelman

Hyaluronic Acid and Its Degradation Products Modulate
Angiogenesis In Vivo and In Vitro 90
S. Kumar and D. West

Inhibitors of Angiogenesis: Angiostatic Steroids 95
J. Folkman and D.E. Ingber

Regulation of Metalloproteinase Activity By
Microvascular Endothelial Cells 101
M.J. Banda, G.S. Herron, G. Murphy, and Z. Werb

Studies on the Regulation of Protease Activity during Cell Invasion and Angiogenesis   110
D.B. Rifkin, O. Saksela, D. Moscatelli, M. Presta,
P. Mignatti, and L. Ossowski

Retinal Pigment Epithelial Cells Release Inhibitors of Neovascularization   114
B.M. Glaser, P.A. Campochiaro, J.L. Davis, Jr., and
J. Jerdan

Inhibitors of Endothelial Cell Proliferation   119
P. Böhlen, M. Fràter-Schroeder, T. Michel, and
Z.-P. Jiang

The Role of the Pericyte in Microvascular Growth Control   125
P.A. D'Amore and A. Orlidge

Differential Angiogenesis   131
R. Auerbach

Regulation of Embryonic Blood Vessel Development   134
W. Risau, R. Hallmann, H. Sariola, P. Ekblom,
R. Kemler, and T. Doetschman

Proliferation and Migration of Irradiated Endothelial Cells   139
M.M. Sholley and J.D. Wilson

Growth Factors Recruit Cells and Modulate Collagen Degradation in Wound Repair and Human Skin Fibroblasts   145
J.M. Davidson, A. Buckley, S.C. Woodward, R.M. Senior,
G.L. Griffin, and M. Klagsbrun

Environmental Regulation of Macrophage Angiogenesis   150
D. Knighton, S. Schumerth, and V. Fiegel

Angiogenesis Induced by Normal Human Breast Tissue   155
H.M. Jensen

Closing Remarks   159
J. Folkman

Introduction

M. Klagsbrun

Departments of Biological Chemistry and Surgery
Children's Hospital and Harvard Medical School
Boston, Massachusetts 02115

Proliferation of blood vessels is a process necessary for the normal growth and development of tissue. In the adult, angiogenesis occurs infrequently. Exceptions are found in the female reproductive system, where angiogenesis occurs in the follicle during its development, in the corpus luteum during ovulation, and in the placenta after pregnancy. These periods of angiogenesis are relatively brief and tightly regulated. Normal angiogenesis also occurs as part of the body's repair processes, e.g., in the healing of wounds and fractures. In contrast, uncontrolled angiogenesis can contribute to serious disease. As examples, the growth of solid tumors is dependent on vascularization and, in diabetic retinopathy, vascularizaton of the retina often leads to blindness.

Some of the earliest insights into the mechanisms of angiogenesis came from studies of tumor vascularization. Experiments with tumors implanted into transparent chambers suggested that the growth of solid tumors was accompanied by new capillary growth. Furthermore, it was demonstrated that tumor cells separated from the vascular bed of a host by a Millipore filter induced the growth of new capillaries. These results suggested that tumor-derived diffusible factors were responsible for stimulating blood vessel growth in the host. Thus, the concept of tumor angiogenesis factors was introduced. Subsequently, it was found that angiogenesis factors could be isolated from normal tissue as well.

Angiogenesis Assays

In order to purify putative angiogenesis factors, in vitro and in vivo bioassays were developed. The in vitro assays were based on steps in capillary growth that could be recapitulated in vitro. New capillaries arise as offshoots or sprouts from established vessels, mostly venules or other capillaries. This phenomenon of capillary sprouting is accomplished by a series of sequential steps. In the initial phase of capillary sprouting, the basement membrane of endothelial cells in the parent blood vessel is degraded. Degradation of the basement membrane is probably accomplished by the action of proteolytic enzymes endogenous to endothelial cells that are induced by angiogenesis factors, most

1

notably plasminogen activator and collagenase. Once the basement membrane is degraded, endothelial cells bud out from the preexisting vessel and migrate directionally into the perivascular space. Cells that have migrated out of the parent blood vessel proliferate so as to elongate the budding sprout. Subsequently, the endothelial cells form tubes containing a lumen through which blood flows. As a final step, new basement membrane is synthesized and a mature new capillary is established. Induction of steps in capillary development, such as endothelial cell locomotion, proliferation, and protease production, has been used as the basis of in vitro bioassays. Three types of assays that have been used are as follows: (1) The induction of endothelial cell migration is assayed either by measuring endothelial cell motility (chemokinesis) using the phagokinetic track assay or by measuring directional endothelial cell migration in a concentration gradient (chemotaxis) using a Boyden migration chamber; (2) the induction of endothelial cell proliferation is assayed either by counting cell number or by monitoring [^{3}H]thymidine uptake into DNA; and (3) the induction of endothelial protease activity is measured by assaying plasminogen activator and latent collagenase.

The two most commonly used bioassays for measuring angiogenesis in vivo are the developing chick chorioallantoic membrane (CAM) and the corneal implant. The CAM bioassay is carried out either in an egg in which a window is prepared by removing a piece of eggshell or by totally removing the shell and culturing the egg in a petri dish. Test substances are applied to filters or plastic coverslips or are incorporated into methylcellulose pellets that are subsequently placed onto an 8–10-day-old CAM. Neovascularization at the site of implant is monitored visually for 1–2 days, and after fixation, CAMs are evaluated histologically. The most reliable bioassay for angiogenesis uses the avascular cornea of either the rabbit or rat eye. Test substances are incorporated into sustained-release polymer pellets, which are implanted into a pocket prepared in the cornea surgically. In a positive angiogenesis response, the directional growth of new capillaries from the limbal blood vessels toward the implant is seen after 5–6 days. In controls, the cornea remains avascular. The corneal bioassay can be quantitated by measuring the rate of blood vessel growth and the density of the new blood vessels.

These in vitro and in vivo assays have been used to identify and isolate a number of angiogenesis factors from both tumors and normal tissue. Some of these angiogenesis factors have been purified, their primary amino acid sequences have been determined, and their genes have been cloned. Other angiogenesis factors have been only partially purified.

Fibroblast Growth Factors—A Family of Heparin-binding Endothelial Cell Mitogens

One strategy in the purification of angiogenesis factors has been to isolate growth factors that stimulate endothelial cell motility and proliferation in vitro. The rationale is that growth factors that stimulate endothelial cell migration and proliferation, key components in capillary growth and development, might be angiogenic in vivo. Among the first endothelial cell growth factors (ECGFs) to be identified were a basic fibroblast growth factor (FGF) isolated from brain and an ECGF isolated from hypothalamus. Other sources of ECGF were retina, eye, and cartilage. A major advance in purifiying ECGFs came as a result of the observation that an ECGF derived from rat chondrosarcoma had a marked affinity for heparin. A rapid two-step procedure combining cation exchange chromatography and heparin-Sepharose chromatography was used to purify a cationic 18,000-molecular-weight chondrosarcoma-derived growth factor to homogeneity. Subsequently, it was found that many, if not all, ECGFs had a marked affinity for heparin and that heparin affinity chromatography could be used to purify a variety of ECGFs, including those found in brain, pituitary, hypothalamus, eye, and cartilage. With the availability of homogeneous growth factor, it was possible for the first time in 1985 to obtain primary amino acid sequences of ECGFs. The first reported primary amino acid sequences were those of bovine brain and pituitary basic FGFs (bFGFs), identical polypeptides of 146 amino acids, and of bovine brain acidic FGF (aFGF), a polypeptide of 140 amino acids. bFGF and aFGF were found to be structurally related, having a 53% absolute sequence homology.

Analysis of the various heparin-binding ECGFs by heparin affinity column elution profiles, protein sequences, immunological cross-reactivity, and receptor binding has greatly clarified the relationship of these polypeptides to one another. There are not as many different ECGFs as previously thought. In fact, most ECGFs can be subdivided into two classes, one containing growth factors structurally related to aFGF and the other, to bFGF. The growth factors within a given class either are identical or represent multiple molecular-weight forms of the same polypeptide.

The class of aFGF consists of anionic polypeptides that elute from heparin-Sepharose columns with approximately 1.0 M NaCl. They have isoelectric points of 5–7 and molecular weights of 15,000–19,000. The aFGF class of heparin-binding growth factors has been found mainly in neural tissue and includes brain-derived aFGF, hypothalmus-derived ECGF, eye-derived growth factor II, retina-derived growth factor, astroglial growth factor-1, and a bone-derived growth factor.

3

The other class of heparin-binding endothelial cell mitogens consists of cationic polypeptides that elute from heparin-Sepharose at approximately 1.5 M NaCl. They have isoelectric points of 8–10 and molecular weights between 16,000 and 19,000, and they appear to be identical to, or multiple molecular-weight forms of, bFGF. The cationic class of heparin-binding growth factor appears to be far more ubiquitous than the anionic class. Polypeptides of this class have been isolated from sources such as pituitary, brain, hypothalamus, eye, cartilage, bone, corpus luteum, adrenal cortex, kidney, placenta, macrophages, chondrosarcoma, hepatoma cells, endothelial cells, astroglial cells, and developing brain. bFGF produced by cultured cells such as hepatoma and endothelial cells appears not to be secreted.

The availability of aFGF and bFGF primary amino acid sequences has resulted in the cloning of aFGF and bFGF genes. A human complementary DNA (cDNA) clone encoding ECGF, a precursor of aFGF, has been isolated from a human-brain-stem cDNA library, and a bovine cDNA clone encoding bFGF has been isolated from a pituitary cDNA library. In both genes, the predicted amino acid sequences of the open reading frame begin with a methionine start codon followed by 154 amino acids. There appear to be no classic signal peptide domains in either the ECGF or bFGF gene, consistent with the lack of secretion of these factors by cultured cells. Structural studies indicate that aFGF and bFGF are 154 amino acid polypeptides in agreement with the gene sequences. The shorter forms of aFGF (140 amino acids) and bFGF (146 amino acids) that were originally isolated and sequenced were truncated forms produced by proteolytic cleavage at the amino-terminal end.

Heparin-binding growth factors not only stimulate endothelial cell proliferation in vitro at about 1 ng/ml, but are angiogenic in vivo as well. bFGF and aFGF in nanogram amounts induce angiogenesis in the CAM, in the cornea, and in wound-healing models. Their angiogenic potential is probably related to their ability to stimulate the migration and proliferation of endothelial cells.

Angiogenin

Angiogenin was first purified from the conditioned medium of a human adenocarcinoma cell line. Angiogenin is a single-chain polypeptide of 123 amino acids with a molecular weight of 14,400 and an isoelectric point of 9.5. Angiogenin has a 35% absolute sequence homology with a family of pancreatic ribonucleases. The major active-site residues of ribonuclease in angiogenin are conserved, as are three of the four disulfide bonds. Angiogenin is inactive toward the more conventional substrates of ribonuclease, such as wheat germ RNA, poly(C), poly(U), and RNA-DNA hybrids. However, angiogenin does cleave both 28S and 18S ribosomal RNAs to relatively large products that are 100–500 nucleotides in length. Whether this relatively specific hydrolytic activity has physiological significance is not known at this time. Angiogenin is a potent stimulator of angiogenesis in the range of 0.5–290 ng/egg in the chick CAM and 50 ng/eye in the rabbit cornea. Although both angiogenin and the heparin-binding growth factors are potent angiogenic factors, they are unrelated molecules. They differ in that (1) angiogenin lacks sequence homology with either aFGF or bFGF; (2) angiogenin does not bind to heparin-Sepharose; (3) angiogenin is secreted by cultured cells, unlike FGF; and (4) angiogenin does not appear to be a growth factor for endothelial cells. In all, these results suggest that angiogenin and the family of heparin-binding ECGFs stimulate angiogenesis via different mechanisms, which have yet to be elucidated.

Transforming Growth Factors
Transforming growth factors (TGFs) are polypeptides that alter the phenotype of normal cells to that of transformed cells. These polypeptides are also capable of inducing angiogenesis in vivo. Two structurally distinct TGFs, TGF-α and TGF-β, have been purified, and their structures have been determined by protein sequencing and cDNA cloning. TGF-α is a 50-amino-acid polypeptide, synthesized by various transformed cells, that binds to the epidermal growth factor (EGF) receptor and has a 35% sequence homology with EGF. Both TGF-α and EGF stimulate microvascular endothelial cell proliferation at 1–5 ng/ml. When these polypeptides are injected subcutaneously into the hamster cheek pouch, they both stimulate capillary proliferation and an increase in the labeling index of endothelial cells. However, TGF-α is a more potent angiogenic factor, being angiogenic at a dose of 0.3–1 μg; whereas, EGF is angiogenic only at a dose of 10 μg.

TGF-β is a 25,000-molecular-weight homodimer found in tumors and normal tissue cells such as placenta, kidney, and platelets. When injected subcutaneously into newborn mice, TGF-β, at a dose of 1 μg, stimulates angiogenesis and collagen production by fibroblasts to form a highly vascular granulation tissue at the site of injection in 2–3 days. Neither EGF nor platelet-derived growth factor has the same effect in the same bioassay. Paradoxically, TGF-β inhibits the growth of aortic endothelial cells in vitro. It is difficult at this point to reconcile the angiogenic activity of TGF-β in vivo with its inhibitory effects on endothelial cell growth in vitro.

5

Chemotactic Factors

Angiogenesis factors that stimulate the locomotion, but not the proliferation, of endothelial cells have been isolated from wound fluid. These factors appear to be polypeptides with molecular weights in the range of 2,000 to 14,000 but have yet to be purified. The material induces angiogenesis in the cornea at a dose of 150 ng. The wound-fluid-derived angiogenesis factors stimulate the migration of capillary endothelial cells in a Boyden chamber assay but do not stimulate the proliferation of these cells. It is possible that these factors are responsible for the endothelial migration component of angiogenesis and that mitogens in wound fluid, perhaps synthesized by macrophages, are responsible for capillary growth and elongation.

Lipids

Several angiogenesis factors that are lipid rather than peptide in nature have been described. 3T3 cells that have undergone adipose differentiation in vitro secrete factors that stimulate angiogenesis in the CAM. These factors stimulate the motility of aortic and capillary endothelial cells in a Boyden chamber assay, but not the proliferation of these cells. Characterization of the angiogenesis/chemotactic factors, including chemical analysis and the use of inhibitors of prostaglandin synthesis, suggests that they may be a mixture of prostaglandins E_1 and E_2 (PGE_1 and PGE_2) and as yet uncharacterized polar lipids. Separate factors that stimulate endothelial cell proliferation, but not endothelial cell motility, are also produced by differentiated 3T3 cells. These endothelial cell mitogens apparently are not lipids, but their identity has not yet been determined.

Prostaglandins, in particular PGE_1 and PGE_2, have been shown to directly stimulate angiogenesis. PGE_1 at 1 μg will stimulate angiogenesis in the cornea, and PGE_2 at 0.2–20 ng will stimulate angiogenesis in the CAM. Other prostaglandins, e.g., the A or F series, are not angiogenic. Prostaglandin levels are elevated in tumors, activated macrophages, wounds, and inflammatory exudates. Since these cells and fluids are associated with neovascularization, it may well be that certain prostaglandins play a role in angiogenesis.

A lipid angiogenic factor extractable in chloroform-methanol has been isolated from omentum. When this material is injected directly into the cornea, intense vascularization occurs. The omentum-derived angiogenesis factor has not yet been purified.

Tumor-derived Low-molecular-weight Angiogenesis Factors

Low-molecular-weight compounds, ranging from 200 to 1000, that stimulate endothelial cell proliferation and angiogenesis in the CAM and cornea have been isolated from Walker 256 tumors. Similar factors have been found in synovial fluid. These factors appear to be neither peptide, protein, nucleic acid, or prostaglandin, and their purification has not yet been accomplished.

Mechanisms of Angiogenesis

It is clear that there are a number of different factors that are capable of stimulating angiogenesis in vivo. Some of these, such as aFGF, bFGF, angiogenin, TGF-α, and TGF-β, have been purified and sequenced, and their genes have been cloned. Others have yet to be fully purified. Although all of these factors are angiogenic in vivo, their effects on endothelial cell motility and proliferation in vitro vary. For example, although aFGF and bFGF are mitogenic for endothelial cells, angiogenin appears not to be mitogenic for these cells and TGF-β is actually an inhibitor of endothelial cell proliferation. Some angiogenic factors, such as aFGF and bFGF, stimulate both endothelial cell motility and proliferation. Others, however, such as the wound-derived angiogenesis factor and the 3T3-adipocyte lipid angiogenesis factors, are chemotactic but not mitogenic for endothelial cells. These results suggest that the various angiogenesis factors might act via different mechanisms. One possibility is that angiogenesis factors act either directly or indirectly to stimulate capillary growth. Some angiogenesis factor mechanisms that have been suggested are as follows: (1) They might act by directly stimulating endothelial cell motility and proliferation, two key events in blood vessel growth and development. (2) They might act directly to stimulate endothelial cell motility alone but induce the total angiogenic response by positioning endothelial cells so that they can be stimulated to proliferate by mitogenic factors. (3) They might act indirectly by mobilizing secondary cells to produce angiogenesis factors that stimulate endothelial cells to migrate and proliferate. A good candidate for an angiogenic secondary cell is the macrophage that produces both bFGF and an angiogenic factor chemotactic but not mitogenic for endothelial cells. (4) They might act indirectly by stimulating endothelial cells to produce their own angiogenesis factors, which could be released to stimulate endothelial cell growth in an autocrine manner. (5) They might act indirectly by liberating angiogenesis factors that are stored in tissue. As an example, bFGF has been found to be stored in the extracellular matrix of aortic and corneal endothelial cells grown in vitro and in Descemet's membrane, the basement membrane produced by the cornea in vivo.

At present, there is not enough evidence to ascertain which of the various angiogenesis factors are acting by direct or indirect mechanisms. bFGF, which is produced by tumors, normal tissue capable of

7

intense angiogenesis (e.g., corpus luteum and placental), and macrophages, and which is stored in basement membrane, is a good candidate for being a factor responsible for direct angiogenesis. On the other hand, non-endothelial cell mitogens, such as TGF-β, angiogenin, and lipid angiogenesis factors, are good candidates for being indirect angiogenesis factors.

Regulation of Angiogenesis

The ubiquity of angiogenesis factors such as bFGF suggests that they must be tightly regulated under normal conditions. For example, considerable quantities of angiogenic ECGF are found in normal tissues, yet the vascular endothelial cell turnover time in most normal tissues is measured in years. Certain cells and tissues, such as lymphocytes and ovary, display brief angiogenesis but then return to the quiescent state. In contrast, the vascular endothelial cells within a tumor are maximally proliferating. Their turnover time is measured in days. There may be many ways to regulate angiogenesis activity. Possible regulatory mechanisms include (1) controlled expression of angiogenesis genes, (2) processing and posttranslational modification of angiogenesis factors, (3) sequestering of angiogenesis factors so that they are not available, (4) controlled release of angiogenesis factors from cells and tissue, and (5) interaction of angiogenesis stimulators with specific angiogenesis inhibitors. Abnormal angiogenesis, such as occurs in tumors and diabetic retinopathy, might be the result of the breakdown of some of these postulated regulatory mechanisms.

Future Directions

The rapid progress of the last 2 years in purifying angiogenesis factors and cloning their genes promises to lead angiogenesis research into important new directions, such as (1) identification of which cells are producers of angiogenesis factors and which are targets, (2) elucidation of how angiogenesis factors are regulated, (3) elucidation of the mechanisms by which angiogenesis factors act, (4) purification of angiogenesis inhibitors, (5) modulation of angiogenesis activity, (6) administration of angiogenesis factors in vivo in order to repair damaged tissue such as occurs in myocardial infarctions, wounds, and bone fractures, and (7) suppression of pathological angiogenesis such as occurs in tumors, diabetic retinopathy, and rheumatoid arthritis.

The papers in this volume cover some of the most recent research in the angiogenesis field. The topics include angiogenesis factors, angiogenesis inhibitors, the biology of endothelial cells, and the biology of angiogenesis in vivo.

8

Structure and Activities of Acidic Fibroblast Growth Factor

K. Thomas, G. Gimenez-Gallego, J. DiSalvo, D. Linemeyer, L. Kelly, J. Menke, T. Mellin, and R. Busch

Department of Biochemistry and Molecular Biology
Merck Sharp and Dohme Research Laboratories
Rahway, New Jersey 07065

Fibroblast growth factor (FGF) activity was originally described in crude brain homogenates almost 50 years ago and was later shown to be present in pituitary tissue (for review, see Thomas and Gimenez-Gallego 1986). In the 1970s, D. Gospodarowicz and colleagues partially purified FGFs from both of these tissues. At least a part of the fibroblast mitogenic activity of these extracts can now be attributed to two related proteins, acidic FGF (aFGF) and basic FGF (bFGF). Both FGFs have been purified to homogeneity (Lemmon and Bradshaw 1983; Bohlen et al. 1984; Thomas et al. 1984). They have subsequently been purified under a variety of different names (heparin-binding growth factors, endothelial cell growth factor, eye-derived growth factors, retina-derived growth factors, astroglial growth factors, etc.) reflecting their sources, targets, and avid binding to heparin-Sepharose (Shing et al. 1984).

Structure and Homologies of FGFs

We have purified to apparent homogeneity (Thomas et al. 1984; Gimenez-Gallego et al. 1986a) and completed the amino acid sequences of both bovine (Gimenez-Gallego et al. 1985) and human (Gimenez-Gallego et al. 1986b) aFGFs. As expected, the bovine and human aFGFs are very similar, having only 11 differences between their 140-residue sequences. Figure 1 shows that a strong homology also exists between acidic and basic FGFs (Esch et al. 1985; Gimenez-Gallego et al. 1985; Thomas and Gimenez-Gallego 1986). As aligned, these two FGFs are about 55% identical in their sequences. A weaker similarity is also detectable between the FGFs and the lymphokine interleukin-1s (IL-1s). As shown in Figure 1, the biologically active carboxy-terminal halves of the IL-1 precursors align with the FGFs.

9

```
AFGF
BFGF    PRO      -ALA-LEU-PRO-GLU-ASP-GLY-GLY-              PHE ASN    -LEU-PRO-
IL-1B   VAL-HIS-ASP-ALA-PRO-VAL-ARG-                       SER GLY-ALA-  -PHE-PRO-
IL-1A   PRO-ARG-SER-ALA-PRO-PHE-SER-PHE-LEU-SER-ASN-VAL-LYS-TYR ASN PHE-MET-ARG-
                                                           SER LEU ASN    -CYS-THR-


AFGF    -LEU-GLY ASN TYR-LYS          -LYS PRO-LYS LEU LEU          TYR-CYS-
BFGF    -PRO GLY HIS-PHE LYS          -ASP PRO-LYS ARG LEU          TYR-CYS-
IL-1B   LEU ARG-ASP-SER-GLN-           -GLN    LYS SER LEU           -VAL-MET-
IL-1A   -ILE-ILE-LYS TYR GLU-PHE-ILE-LEU-ASN-   -ASP-ALA LEU ASN-GLN-SER-ILE-ILE-


AFGF     SER     ASN-GLY-GLY  TYR PHE   LEU-ARG-ILE-LEU-PRO-ASP-GLY THR VAL-ASP-
BFGF    -LYS-    ASN-GLY-GLY  PHE PHE   LEU-ARG-ILE HIS PRO-ASP-GLY ARG VAL-ASP-
IL-1B    SER          GLY PRO TYR GLU-  LEU LYS ALA-LEU-HIS LEU-GLN-GLY-GLN ASP
IL-1A   -ARG-ALA ASN ASP-GLN TYR LEU-THR-ALA-ALA ALA-LEU-HIS ASN-LEU-ASP-GLU-ALA-


AFGF     GLY                                   -THR-LYS-ASP-ARG SER-ASP
BFGF     GLY                                   -VAL-ARG GLU-LYS-SER-ASP
IL-1B   -MET-GLU-GLN-GLN-VAL-VAL PHE SER MET SER-PHE-VAL-GLN-GLY GLU GLU SER ASN
IL-1A   -VAL-LYS-              PHE ASP MET GLY-ALA-TYR-LYS-SER-SER LYS ASP ASP


AFGF     GLN HIS-ILE GLN LEU-GLN-LEU CYS ALA-GLU SER-ILE GLY GLU VAL-TYR-ILE-
BFGF    -PRO HIS-ILE LYS LEU-GLN-LEU GLN ALA-GLU-GLU ARG GLY VAL VAL SER ILE-
IL-1B   -ASP LYS ILE PRO VAL ALA LEU-GLY-LEU-LYS GLU    -LYS-ASN LEU-TYR LEU-SER-
IL-1A   -ALA LYS ILE THR VAL ILE LEU-ARG-ILE-SER-LYS-   -THR-GLN LEU-TYR VAL-THR-


AFGF             -LYS SER-THR-GLU-THR-GLY-GLN-PHE LEU-ALA-MET ASP-THR ASP-GLY
BFGF             -LYS GLY-VAL-CYS-ALA-ASN-ARG-TYR LEU-ALA-MET LYS GLU-ASP-GLY
IL-1B   -CYS-VAL-LEU LYS ASP ASP LYS PRO THR LEU GLN LEU GLU    -SER-VAL ASP PRO-
IL-1A      -ALA-GLN-ASP-GLU ASP GLN PRO VAL LEU LEU-LYS GLU MET PRO GLU ILE PRO-


AFGF    -LEU LEU TYR GLY SER GLN-THR-PRO ASN-GLU-GLU-CYS LEU PHE LEU GLU-ARG-LEU-
BFGF    -ARG LEU LEU-ALA SER LYS CYS-VAL-THR-ASP GLU-CYS-PHE PHE PHE GLU-ARG-LEU-
IL-1B   -LYS ASN TYR PRO-    LYS LYS-LYS-MET GLU LYS-ARG PHE VAL PHE ASN-LYS-ILE-
IL-1A   -LYS THR-ILE-THR-GLY-SER-GLU-THR ASN LEU-LEU-  PHE-PHE TRP GLU THR-HIS-


AFGF    -GLU GLU ASN HIS TYR-ASN-THR-TYR ILE SER LYS LYS-HIS ALA-GLU-LYS-HIS TRP
BFGF    -GLU SER ASN-ASN-TYR-ASN-THR-TYR ARG SER ARG LYS TYR-SER-    SER TRP-
IL-1B   GLU ILE ASN-ASN LYS-LEU-GLU PHE GLU SER ALA-GLN-PHE PRO-     -ASN TRP-
IL-1A   -GLY-THR-LYS ASN-TYR-      -PHE THR SER VAL-ALA HIS-PRO-      -ASN LEU-


AFGF     PHE-VAL GLY LEU-LYS LYS-ASN GLY ARG-SER LYS-     -LEU-GLY PRO ARG THR
BFGF    -TYR VAL-ALA-LEU-LYS ARG-THR GLY GLN-TYR LYS-     -LEU-GLY PRO LYS THR
IL-1B   -TYR ILE SER THR SER GLN ALA-GLU-ASN-MET-PRO-VAL-PHE LEU-GLY-GLY    THR
IL-1A   PHE-ILE-ALA-THR LYS GLN ASP-TYR-TRP-VAL-    -CYS LEU ALA GLY


AFGF    -HIS-PHE GLY-GLN-LYS-ALA-ILE-LEU-  -PHE-LEU-PRO-LEU PRO VAL-SER-SER ASP
BFGF    -GLY-PRO GLY-GLN-LYS-ALA-ILE-LEU-  -PHE-LEU-PRO MET-SER-ALA-LYS SER
IL-1B   -LYS-GLY GLY-GLN ASP-    ILE THR-ASP PHE THR-MET-GLN-PHE VAL-SER-SER
IL-1A      GLY PRO-PRO-SER ILE THR-ASP PHE GLN-ILE LEU GLU-ASN-GLN-ALA
```

Figure 1 *(See facing page for legend.)*

10

From analysis of sequence homology alone, the FGFs and IL-1s are related to each other with a significance of about 2 standard deviations from random. By hydropathicity analysis, a method of detecting similarities in distantly related proteins, the FGFs and IL-1s are related to each other with a significance of about 6 standard deviations from random (Gimenez-Gallego et al. 1985). We infer from these data that the FGFs and IL-1s have similar three-dimensional polypeptide folding patterns. Therefore, the FGFs and IL-1s appear to define a new class of homologous growth factors that diverged from a common ancestral protein.

Biological Activities

aFGF is a mitogen for a variety of cells in culture, including large vessel and microvascular endothelial cells, chondrocytes, myoblasts, osteoblasts, and glial cells. Heparin appears to stabilize or activate aFGF to varying degrees, depending on the method of purification, conditions of storage, and/or the particular cell culture used to monitor activity (Gimenez-Gallego et al. 1986a). In vivo, pure aFGF is angiogenic on the chick egg chorioallantoic membrane (Thomas et al. 1985), an activity that is augmented about fourfold by heparin (Lobb et al. 1985). The mitogen is also angiogenic in a hamster cheek pouch assay at 300 ng/animal in the absence of heparin (A.B. Schreiber and K. Thomas, unpubl.).

A synthetic gene for bovine aFGF has been constructed from 16 long oligonucleotides and expressed in *Escherichia coli*. Recombinant aFGF has been purified to homogeneity by a two-step procedure using heparin-Sepharose and C_4 reversed-phase high-performance liquid chromatography and shown to be highly active in a BALB/c-3T3 mitogenesis assay. Both brain-derived and recombinant aFGFs were tested for their ability to accelerate the rate of dermal wound healing in mice. Punch biopsies were made through the epidermis and dermis. The wounds were treated twice daily either with 500 ng/dose of aFGF containing 2 μg of heparin or with heparin controls. Wound surface areas were recorded daily. Heparin alone had no effect on wound

Figure 1 Amino acid sequences of FGFs and homologies with IL-1s. The complete amino acid sequences of bovine brain-derived aFGF (AFGF) and pituitary-derived bFGF (BFGF) are aligned with the carboxy-terminal halves of the precursors of both human IL-1β (IL-1B) and IL-1α (IL-1A) beginning at residues 114 and 110, respectively. The amino terminus of IL-1β starts at Ala-117. Mature mouse IL-1α starts at a position equivalent to Ser-112 in the human protein. Common aligned residues are enclosed in boxes. (Reprinted, with permission, from Thomas and Gimenez-Gallego 1986.)

11

closure. The combination of aFGF with heparin, however, significantly accelerated the rate at which the wounds closed. On the basis of this activity, aFGF might be useful as a therapeutic agent in humans.

REFERENCES

Bohlen, P., A. Baird, F. Esch, N. Ling, and D. Gospodarowicz. 1984. Isolation and partial characterization of pituitary fibroblast growth factor. *Proc. Natl. Acad. Sci.* **81**: 5364.

Esch, F., A. Baird, N. Ling, N. Ueno, F. Hill, L. Denoroy, R. Klepper, D. Gospodarowicz, P. Bohlen, and R. Guillemin. 1985. Primary structure of bovine pituitary basic fibroblast growth factor (FGF) and comparison with the amino-terminal sequence of bovine acidic FGF. *Proc. Natl. Acad. Sci.* **82**: 6507.

Gimenez-Gallego, G., G. Conn, V.B. Hatcher, and K.A. Thomas. 1986a. Human brain-derived acidic fibroblast growth factors: Amino terminal sequences and specific mitogenic activities. *Biochem. Biophys. Res. Commun.* **135**: 541.

―――. 1986b. The complete amino acid sequence of human brain-derived acidic fibroblast growth factor. *Biochem. Biophys. Res. Commun.* **138**: 611.

Gimenez-Gallego, G., J. Rodkey, C. Bennett, M. Rios-Candelore, J. DiSalvo, and K. Thomas. 1985. Brain-derived acidic fibroblast growth factor: Complete amino acid sequence and homologies. *Science* **230**: 1385.

Lemmon, S.K. and R.A. Bradshaw. 1983. Purification and partial characterization of bovine pituitary fibroblast growth factor. *J. Cell. Biochem.* **21**: 195.

Lobb, R.R., E.M. Alderman, and J.W. Fett. 1985. Induction of angiogenesis by bovine brain-derived class 1 heparin-binding growth factor. *Biochemistry* **24**: 4969.

Shing, Y., J. Folkman, R. Sullivan, C. Butterfield, J. Murray, and M. Klagsbrun. 1984. Heparin affinity: Purification of a tumor-derived capillary endothelial cell growth factor. *Science* **223**: 1296.

Thomas, K.A. and G. Gimenez-Gallego. 1986. Fibroblast growth factors: Broad spectrum mitogens with potent angiogenic activity. *Trends Biochem. Sci.* **11**: 81.

Thomas, K.A., M. Rios-Candelore, and S. Fitzpatrick. 1984. Purification and characterization of acidic fibroblast growth factor from bovine brain. *Proc. Natl. Acad. Sci.* **81**: 357.

Thomas, K.A., M. Rios-Candelore, G. Gimenez-Gallego, J. DiSalvo, C. Bennett, J. Rodkey, and S. Fitzpatrick. 1985. Pure brain-derived acidic fibroblast growth factor is a potent angiogenic vascular endothelial cell mitogen with sequence homology to interleukin 1. *Proc. Natl. Acad. Sci.* **82**: 6409.

Multiple Forms of Hepatoma-derived Basic Fibroblast Growth Factor: Cleavages by Tumor Cell Acid Proteinases

M. Klagsbrun

Departments of Biological Chemistry and Surgery
Children's Hospital and Harvard Medical School
Boston, Massachusetts 02115

A strong affinity for heparin is a characteristic of most, if not all, endothelial cell growth factors. Comparative structural analysis of these polypeptides suggests that the heparin-binding endothelial cell growth factors fall into two classes whose prototypes are acidic and basic fibroblast growth factors (FGFs) (Lobb et al. 1986). Basic FGF (bFGF) derived from brain and pituitary cells has been sequenced and shown to be a polypeptide of 146 amino acids (Esch et al. 1985). We recently purified an endothelial cell growth factor, synthesized by human hepatoma cells, that was immunologically and structurally related to bFGF (Klagsbrun et al. 1986). However, the hepatoma-derived bFGF differed from bovine brain and pituitary bFGFs in that it appeared to be a higher-molecular-weight form of bFGF extended at the amino terminus. Lower-molecular-weight forms of bFGF missing 15 amino acids from the amino terminus have also been isolated, for example, from corpus luteum, kidney, and adrenal gland (Baird et al. 1985; Gospodarowicz et al. 1985, 1986). The existence of at least three discrete molecular-weight forms of bFGF suggests that this polypeptide might be proteolytically processed in cells and tissues.

Multiple Forms of Hepatoma-derived bFGF

The 146-amino-acid form of bFGF was purified after extraction of brain and pituitary cells at acid pH (Esch et al. 1985), and the higher-molecular-weight form of bFGF synthesized by hepatoma cells was purified after extraction of cells at neutral pH (Klagsbrun et al. 1986). These results suggested that extraction at acid pH might affect the molecular weight of bFGF. To ascertain whether the pH of extraction was a variable in determining molecular weight, bFGF was extracted

13

from hepatoma cells by two methods, at acid pH (Gospodarowicz et al. 1978) and at neutral pII (Klagsbrun et al. 1986). After extraction, hepatoma cell bFGF was purified and analyzed by SDS-PAGE (Fig. 1). Hepatoma bFGF purified after extraction at neutral pH had a molecular weight of about 18,400. On the other hand, acid pH extraction of hepatoma cells yielded two lower-molecular-weight forms of bFGF: a minor species with a molecular weight of approximately 17,500 and a major species with a molecular weight of approximately 16,500.

The cleavage products of bFGF generated by acid pH extraction were not formed by direct degradation of polypeptide by acid. Both the higher- and lower-molecular-weight forms of bFGF were purified after neutral extraction by a procedure that included reversed-phase liquid chromatography in 0.1% TFA (pH 2). In addition, direct exposure of the 18,400-molecular-weight forms of bFGF to pH 2 for 3 hours at 37°C did not result in growth factor degradation. An alternative explanation for the degradation of bFGF in acid extracts was that they were cleaved by acid proteinases.

Cleavage of Hepatoma Cell bFGF by Acid Proteinases

Homogenates of hepatoma cells were extracted at acid pH in the absence or presence of proteinase inhibitors, and bFGF was subsequently purified and analyzed by SDS-PAGE (Fig. 2). As expected, acid extraction of hepatoma cells produced predominantly the lower-

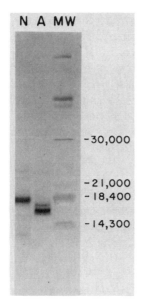

Figure 1 SDS-PAGE analysis of hepatoma bFGF purified after extraction at neutral and acid pH. Hepatoma cells were extracted at either pH 7.0 or pH 4.5. bFGF was purified by a successive combination of BioRex 70, heparin-Sepharose, and reversed-phase liquid chromatography and analyzed by SDS-PAGE and silver stain. (N) bFGF extracted at pH 7.0 (neutral); (A) bFGF extracted at pH 4.5 (acid); (MW) molecular-weight markers.

14

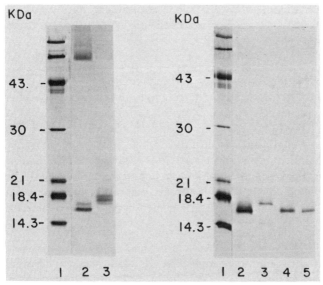

Figure 2 SDS-PAGE analysis of the effects of proteinase inhibitors on the cleavage of hepatoma bFGF. Hepatoma cells were extracted at pH 3.5 with or without proteinase inhibitors, purified, and analyzed by SDS-PAGE and silver staining. (*Left*, Lane *1*) Molecular-weight markers; (*2*) acid pH extraction; (*3*) acid pH extraction in the presence of leupeptin (1 μg/ml), pepstatin (4 μM), and PMSF (1 mM). (*Right*, Lane *1*) Molecular-weight markers; (*2*) acid pH extraction; (*3*) acid pH extraction in the presence of leupeptin; (*4*) acid pH extraction in the presence of pepstatin; (*5*) acid pH extraction in the presence of PMSF.

molecular-weight (16,500) form of bFGF (left panel, lane 2). However, when the acid extracts contained a mixture of pepstatin, leupeptin, and PMSF (left panel, lane 3), degradation was totally inhibited and the higher-molecular-weight (18,400) form was produced. The proteinase inhibitors were tested individually (Fig. 2, right panel). In the presence of leupeptin alone, cleavage to the 16,500-molecular-weight form was inhibited (lane 3). Pepstatin alone (lane 4) and PMSF alone (lane 5) did not inhibit degradation at all.

Electrophoretic Western blots using site-specific antibodies directed against the amino-terminal region, an internal region, and the carboxy-terminal region of bFGF were used to analyze the various molecular-weight forms of hepatoma bFGF. Although the "internal" and "carboxyl" antibodies cross-reacted with the major 16,500-molecular-weight form of bFGF purified after acid pH extraction, the "amino-terminal" antibodies did not. It was concluded that the 16,500-

15

molecular-weight form of bFGF was produced by a cleavage on the amino-terminal end that occurred during acid pH extraction of hepatoma cells.

Growth Factor Activity

Cleavage of hepatoma bFGF at the amino-terminal end by acid protein-ases has no adverse effects on growth factor activity. bFGFs extracted at acid pH (16,500-m.w. form) and at acid pH in the presence of leupeptin, pepstatin, and PMSF (18,400-m.w. form) show the same dose-dependent growth factor activity. Cleavage at the amino-terminal end also does not affect the elution position of bFGF on heparin-Sepharose columns. Thus, it appears that the amino-terminal domain of bFGF is not involved in mitogenicity or in heparin binding.

DISCUSSION

Analysis of the multiple forms of bFGF synthesized by hepatoma cells has led us to the following conclusions: (1) bFGF is actually a larger polypeptide than previously reported. The sequence of brain and pitui-tary bFGF reported by Esch et al. (1985) is that of a truncated 146-amino-acid form (bFGF 1–146) produced by extraction at acid pH and subsequent activation of acid proteinases. (2) An acid proteinase, which is inhibited by leupeptin, is found in hepatoma cells. This enzyme reduces hepatoma cell bFGF from an 18,400-molecular-weight form to a 16,500-molecular-weight form. (3) The acid-proteinase-mediated cleavages occur at the amino terminus of bFGF.

What is the probable size of intact bFGF? The gene for bovine bFGF has recently been cloned (Abraham et al. 1986). An ATG (methionine) codon found nine amino acids upstream of the purported amino-terminal proline (Esch et al. 1985) has been proposed as the start codon. Thus, the nucleotide sequence of bFGF predicts a 155-amino-acid bFGF translation product. Differential amino acid analysis of bFGF extracted at acid pH in the presence and absence of inhibitors has demonstrated the existence of a 154-amino-acid form of bFGF extended by eight residues on the amino-terminal side (Ueno et al. 1986). The identity of the eight residues is consistent with that predict-ed by the bFGF gene, but beyond the initiating methionine. In addi-tion, we have isolated from human hepatoma cells a form of bFGF extended by 17 amino acids on the amino-terminal side and whose amino acid sequence correlates well with the sequence predicted from the human bFGF gene (M. Klagsbrun, unpubl.). Thus, bFGF in some forms might be as large as 163 amino acids. Whether any larger precursors of bFGF exist has yet to be determined.

REFERENCES

Abraham, J.A., A. Mergia, J.L. Whang, A. Tumolo, J. Friedman, K.A. Hjerrild, D. Gospodarowicz, and J.C. Fiddes. 1986. Nucleotide sequence of a bovine clone encoding the angiogenic protein, basic fibroblast growth factor. *Science* **233**: 545.

Baird, A., F. Esch, P. Bohlen, N. Ling, and D. Gospodarowicz. 1985. Isolation and partial characterization of an endothelial cell growth factor from the bovine kidney: Homology with basic fibroblast growth factor. *Regul. Pept.* **12**: 201.

Esch, F., A. Baird, N. Ling, N. Ueno, F. Hill, L. Denoroy, R. Klepper, D. Gospodarowicz, P. Bohlen, and R. Guilleman. 1985. Primary structure of bovine pituitary fibroblast growth factor (FGF) and comparison with the amino-terminal sequence of bovine acidic FGF. *Proc. Natl. Acad. Sci.* **82**: 6507.

Gospodarowicz, D., H. Bialecki, and G. Greenberg. 1978. Purification of the fibroblast growth factor activity from bovine brain. *J. Biol. Chem.* **253**: 3736.

Gospodarowicz, D., A. Baird, J. Cheng, G.M. Lui, F. Esch, and P. Bohlen. 1986. Isolation of fibroblast growth factor from bovine adrenal gland: Physicochemical and biological characteristics. *Endocrinology* **118**: 82.

Gospodarowicz, D., J. Cheng, G.M. Lui, A. Baird, F. Esch, and P. Bohlen. 1985. Corpus luteum angiogenic factor is related to fibroblast growth factor. *Endocrinology* **117**: 2383.

Klagsbrun, M., J. Sasse, R. Sullivan, and J.A. Smith. 1986. Human tumor cells synthesize an endothelial cell growth factor that is structurally related to basic fibroblast growth factor. *Proc. Natl. Acad. Sci.* **83**: 2448.

Lobb, R., J. Sasse, Y. Shing, P. D'Amore, R. Sullivan, J. Jacobs, and M. Klagsbrun. 1986. Purification and characterization of heparin-binding growth factors. *J. Biol. Chem.* **261**: 1924.

Ueno, N., A. Baird, F. Esch, N. Ling, and R. Guillemin. 1986. Isolation of an amino-terminal extended form of basic fibroblast growth factor. *Biochem. Biophys. Res. Commun.* **138**: 580.

17

Endothelial Cell Growth Factor

T. Maciag

Laboratory of Molecular Biology, The Holland Laboratory for
Biomedical Research, American Red Cross, Rockville, Maryland 20855

The process of neovascularization involves an integration of proliferative and nonproliferative biochemical events directed toward the cells that comprise capillary vessels. It is known that the angiogenic process in vivo can be initiated by a rather wide variety of biological response modifiers that include proteolytic enzymes, inorganic ions, members of the arachadonic acid family, and polypeptide growth factors and hormones (Folkman 1974; Folkman and Cotran 1976). The stimulation of neovascularization in vivo by such a diverse set of biochemical response modifiers suggests that this process may be ultimately regulated by a cascade of biochemical events. As a result, it has been proposed that the angiogenic cascade should include multiple levels and a variety of entry and exit points in order to explain the diverse structural nature of known angiogenic factors (Maciag 1984).

To elucidate this pathway, we have concentrated our efforts on defining the structure of a polypeptide growth factor that stimulates the division of human endothelial cells in vitro. Since growth factors, in general, stimulate cell division by the down-regulation of high-affinity cell-surface receptors, we reasoned that, ultimately, the structure of an endothelial cell growth factor (ECGF) would provide information relevant to the mechanism of receptor-mediated angiogenesis (Maciag 1984) and may help to define alternative pathways that are integrated in the angiogenic cascade.

Structure of the Angiogenic Polypeptide ECGF

The acidic polypeptide, ECGF (Maciag et al. 1982), has been purified in relatively large quantities using a rapid purification procedure (Burgess et al. 1986a) that utilizes the relatively high affinity of the polypeptide for the glycosaminoglycan, heparin (Maciag et al. 1984). Two acidic polypeptides were identified and separated by reversed-phase high-pressure liquid chromatography (RP-HPLC) and were named α-ECGF and β-ECGF in reference to the retention time of the polypeptides eluted from RP-HPLC (Burgess et al. 1986a). The complete amino acid sequences of both polypeptides have been determined (Burgess et al. 1986b) and are shown in Figure 1. The sequence

18

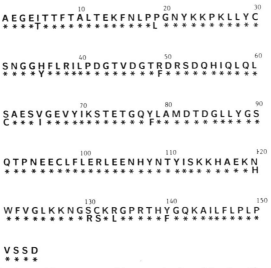

```
              10              20               30
A E G E I T T F T A L T E K F N L P P G N Y K K P K L L Y C
* * * * T * * * * * * * * * * * * * L * * * * * * * * * *

              40              50               60
S N G G H F L R I L P D G T V D G T R D R S D Q H I Q L Q L
* * * * Y * * * ** * * * * * * * F * * * * * * ** * * *

              70              80               90
S A E S V G E V Y I K S T E T G Q Y L A M D T D G L L Y G S
C * * * I * * * ** * * * * * * F ** * * * * ** * * *

              100             110              120
Q T P N E E C L F L E R L E E N H Y N T Y I S K K H A E K N
* * * * * * * * * * * * * * * * * * * ** * * * * * * H

              130             140              150
W F V G L K K N G S C K R G P R T H Y G Q K A I L F L P L P
* * * * * * * * * R S * L ** * * * F * * * * ** * * *

V S S D
* * * *
```

Figure 1 Amino acid sequence of human (*top*) and bovine (*bottom*) ECGF. The human sequence was deduced from the cDNA sequence (Jaye et al. 1986) and the bovine sequence was obtained by protein chemistry methods (Burgess et al. 1986b).

information demonstrates that β-ECGF, the larger of the two polypeptides, contains a blocked amino terminus. The data also suggest that β-ECGF is the polypeptide precursor of α-ECGF. Thus, α-ECGF is the des 1-20 form of β-ECGF. Likewise, the structure of β-ECGF also encompasses the sequence reported for acidic fibroblast growth factor (aFGF), a potent endothelial cell mitogen and stimulator of angiogenesis in vivo (Thomas et al. 1985). Therefore, it is reasonable to suggest that aFGF is the des 1-14 form of β-ECGF. Although the significance of the derivatives of β-ECGF is not known, it is reasonable to suggest that aFGF and α-ECGF are products of the extraction conditions used during the purification procedure and calls attention to the mechanism(s) by which β-ECGF is processed. Whereas cleavage of the K_{14}-F_{15} peptide bond in β-ECGF may involve a serine protease that generates aFGF, cleavage of G_{20}-N_{21} peptide bond in β-ECGF to form α-ECGF is unique (Burgess et al. 1986b).

The Gene Encoding β-ECGF

A human cDNA clone encompassing the open reading frame for β-ECGF was obtained and sequenced (Jaye et al. 1986). The amino acid sequence of the human β-ECGF polypeptide deduced from the cDNA sequence is consistent with the sequence reported for human aFGF

19

(Harper et al. 1986). A comparison of the human and bovine β-ECGF amino acid sequences (Fig. 1) suggests that the gene encoding β-ECGF is highly conserved.

An examination of the nucleotide sequence of the β-ECGF cDNA clone reveals the presence of the sequence, 5'-ACCAUGG-3', that includes a putative initiation codon upstream of the open reading frame (Jaye et al. 1986). This sequence is consistent with the consensus sequence proposed for the initiation of translation in eukaryotes. In addition, the open reading frame is flanked by termination codons, demonstrating that β-ECGF does not contain a preproform. Further examination of the amino acid sequence of β-ECGF reveals the absence of a consensus sequence for a signal peptide.

The apparent absence of a signal peptide for β-ECGF is a feature that it shares with other polypeptide growth factors that are structurally homologous. The amino acid sequence encompassing β-ECGF is approximately 55% homologous to the structure reported for basic FGF (bFGF) (Abraham et al. 1986) and is approximately 30% homologous to the structure reported for interleukin 1 (Jaye et al. 1986). These and other homologies are discussed in detail elsewhere in this volume (for a recent review, see Lobb et al. 1986). The reason for the absence of a signal peptide for these three polypeptide growth factors is presently not known. Although these observations call attention to the potential importance of cell lysis or death as a possible mechanism for growth factor delivery, the mechanism by which ECGF exits a cell must be resolved before a potential autocrine and/or paracrine function for the mitogen can be assigned.

ECGF Receptor

Binding studies performed with the ^{125}I-labeled derivative of α-ECGF demonstrate that endothelial cells and fibroblasts contain high-affinity binding sites present on the cell surface. These cells contain between 20,000 and 40,000 receptors per cell with an average K_d of approximately 1 nM (Schreiber et al. 1985a). A comparison of the K_d for ECGF binding with the concentration of ECGF required to transduce a half-maximum mitogenic signal demonstrates that only partial receptor occupancy is required for biological signal transduction (Schreiber et al. 1985a).

Covalent cross-linking studies with ^{125}I-labeled ECGF have revealed that the high-affinity binding domain present on the surface of endothelial cells is a polypeptide with an M_r of approximately 150,000 (Friesel et al. 1986). The M_r 150,000 ECGF receptor polypeptide is rapidly down-regulated at 37°C but not at 4°C (Friesel et al. 1986), an observation consistent with ligand binding data (Schreiber et al. 1985a).

Ligand binding to the ECGF receptor is prerequisite for mitogenic signal transduction because monoclonal antibodies against ECGF, which bind ECGF but do not inhibit the mitogenic activity of ECGF, do not prevent ^{125}I-labeled ECGF from binding to its receptor. Likewise, monoclonal antibodies that bind ECGF and inhibit the biological activity of ECGF do inhibit the ability of ^{125}I-labeled ECGF to bind to its receptor (Schreiber et al. 1985a).

The binding of brain-derived growth factor I (Huang and Huang 1986), a polypeptide derived from β-ECGF (Burgess et al. 1986b), to its receptor initiates a tyrosine kinase activity at the cell surface that phosphorylates a cross-linked M_r 145,000 polypeptide (Huang and Huang 1986). Although it is presently unclear whether this polypeptide is structurally related to the ECGF receptor, it is likely that these receptors are indeed related. Thus, it is likely that the ECGF receptor may contain an intracellular tyrosine kinase domain that is involved in ECGF-initiated signal transduction.

The Glycosaminoglycan, Heparin, Is a Cofactor for ECGF

The affinity between heparin and ECGF has been used as a basis of distinction between ECGF and other heparin-binding growth factors, bFGF, and platelet-derived growth factor (Lobb et al. 1986). In addition to the avid affinity between ECGF and heparin (Maciag et al. 1984), heparin possesses a number of other unique attributes as a modulator of the biological activity of ECGF. Heparin potentiates the mitogenic activity of crude (Thornton et al. 1984) and pure preparations of ECGF (Schreiber et al. 1984a). In addition, the activity of ECGF as a chemotactic signal for endothelial cell migration is also potentiated by heparin (Terranova et al. 1985). Although the mechanism by which heparin potentiates the biological activities of ECGF is not known, recent studies suggest that heparin may induce in ECGF a favored structural polypeptide conformation.

Evidence for heparin-induced conformational changes include data obtained by immunological and radioreceptor studies (Schreiber et al. 1985a,b). Heparin alters the K_d for ECGF receptor binding and enables monoclonal antibodies prepared against ECGF to bind the antigen with higher affinity (Schreiber et al. 1985a,b). In addition, it is clear that heparin can restore biological activity to preparations of ECGF that have lost considerable potency upon storage (Schreiber et al. 1985a). These data agree with our observation that heparin cannot bind thermally denatured ECGF and may be able to distinguish between native and denatured ECGF conformations (T. Maciag and R. Friesel, unpubl.). However, additional physical evidence is required to establish that these presumed heparin-induced conformational alterations of

ECGF are established by the interaction between the glycosamino-glycan and the polypeptide.

The chemical structure of the glycosaminoglycan present in the preparation of heparin is not known. If one assumes a stoichiometry of 1:1 between the ECGF polypeptide and the glycosaminoglycan, it is reasonable to suggest that a relatively minor component of the heparin preparation is responsible for the cofactor activity. However, it is assumed that the same glycosaminoglycan is responsible for the ECGF-potentiating activities of heparin. Likewise, it is known that heparin, itself, cannot exert a mitogenic effect on endothelial cells in vitro (Thornton et al. 1984; Schreiber et al. 1985a). In contrast, heparin can act as an inhibitor of vascular smooth-muscle-cell proliferation in vitro (Castellot et al. 1981). Although the mechanism of the heparin-induced inhibition of smooth-muscle-cell division is not known, it has been suggested that this event may involve receptor-mediated signal trans-duction. In this regard, it remains to be established whether heparin participates in the mitogenic events induced by ECGF and is internal-ized by ECGF receptor down-regulation as an ECGF:heparin complex.

ACKNOWLEDGMENTS

This is the American Red Cross contribution number 738. Support for this work was provided by National Institutes of Health grants HL-32348 and HL-35627.

REFERENCES

Abraham, J.A., A. Mergia, J.L. Whang, A. Tumolo, J. Friedman, K.A. Hjerrild, D. Gospodarowicz, and J.C. Fiddes. 1986. Nucleotide sequence of a bovine clone encoding the angiogenic protein, basic fibroblast growth factor. *Science* **233**: 545.

Burgess, W.H., T. Mehlman, R. Friesel, W.V. Johnson, and T. Maciag. 1986a. Multiple forms of endothelial cell growth factor. *J. Biol. Chem.* **260**: 11389.

Burgess, W.H., T. Mehlman, D.R. Marshak, B.A. Fraser, and T. Maciag. 1986b. Structural evidence that endothelial cell growth factor β is the precursor of both endothelial cell growth factor α and acidic fibroblast growth factor. *Proc. Natl. Acad. Sci.* **83**: 7216.

Castellot, J.J., M.L. Addonizio, R. Rosenberg, and M.J. Karnovsky. 1981. Cultured endothelial cells produce a heparin-like inhibitor of smooth muscle cell growth. *J. Cell Biol.* **90**: 372.

Friesel, R., W.H. Burgess, T. Mehlman, and T. Maciag. 1986. The characteri-zation of the receptor for endothelial cell growth factor by covalent ligand attachment. *J. Biol. Chem.* **261**: 7581.

Folkman, J. 1963. Angiogenesis. *Adv. Cancer Res.* **7**: 167.

———. 1974. Tumor angiogenesis. *Adv. Cancer Res.* **19**: 331.

Folkman, J. and R. Cotran. 1976. Relation of vascular proliferation to tumor growth. *Int. Rev. Exp. Pathol.* **16**: 207.

Harper, J.W., D.J. Strydom, and R.R. Lobb. 1986. Human class 1 heparin-binding factor: Structure and homology to bovine acidic brain fibroblast growth factor. *Biochemistry* **25**: 4097.

Huang, S.S. and J.F. Huang. 1986. Association of bovine brain-derived growth factor receptor with protein tyrosine kinase activity. *J. Biol. Chem.* **261**: 9568.

Jaye, M., R. Howk, W.H. Burgess, G.A. Ricca, I.-M. Chiu, M. Ravera, S.J. O'Brien, W.S. Modi, T. Maciag, and W.N. Drohan. 1986. Human endothelial cell growth factor: Cloning, nucleotide sequence, and chromosome localization. *Science* **233**: 541.

Lobb, R.R., J.W. Harper, and J.W. Fett. 1986. Purification of heparin-binding growth factors. *Anal. Biochem.* **154**: 1.

Maciag, T. 1984. Angiogenesis. *Prog. Thromb. Hemostasis* **7**: 167.

Maciag, T., G.A. Hoover, and R. Weinstein. 1982. High and low molecular weight forms of endothelial cell growth factor. *J. Biol. Chem.* **257**: 5333.

Maciag, T., T. Mehlman, R. Friesel, and A.B. Schreiber. 1984. Heparin binds endothelial cell-growth factor, the principal endothelial cell mitogen in bovine brain. *Science* **225**: 932.

Schreiber, A.B., J. Kenney, W.J. Kowalski, R. Friesel, T. Mehlman, and T. Maciag. 1985a. Interaction of endothelial cell growth factor with heparin: Characterization by receptor and antibody recognition. *Proc. Natl. Acad. Sci.* **82**: 6138.

Schreiber, A.B., J. Kenney, J. Kowalski, K.A. Thomas, G. Gimenez-Gallego, M. Rios-Candelore, J. DiSalvo, D. Barritault, J. Courty, Y. Courtois, M. Moenner, C. Loret, W.H. Burgess, T. Mehlman, R. Friesel, W.V. Johnson, and T. Maciag. 1985b. A unique family of endothelial cell polypeptide mitogens: The antigenic and receptor cross-reactivity of bovine endothelial cell growth factor, brain-derived acidic fibroblast growth factor, and eye-derived growth factor-II. *J. Cell Biol.* **101**: 1623.

Terranova, V.P., R. DiFlorio, R.M. Lyall, S. Hic, R. Friesel, and T. Maciag. 1985. Human endothelial cells are chemotactic to endothelial-cell growth-factor and heparin. *J. Cell Biol.* **101**: 2330.

Thomas, K.A., M. Rios-Candelore, G. Gimenez-Gallego, J. DiSalvo, C. Bennett, J. Rodkey, and S. Fitzpatrick. 1985. Pure brain-derived acidic fibroblast growth factor is a potent angiogenic vascular endothelial cell mitogen with sequence homology to interleukin 1. *Proc. Natl. Acad. Sci.* **82**: 6409.

Thornton, S.C., S.N. Mueller, and E.M. Levine. 1984. Human endothelial cells: Use of heparin in cloning and long-term serial cultivation. *Science* **222**: 623.

Genes for the Angiogenic Growth Factors: Basic and Acidic Fibroblast Growth Factors

J.C. Fiddes, J.L. Whang, A. Mergia,
A. Tumolo, and J.A. Abraham

California Biotechnology, Inc.
Mountain View, California 94043

Basic and acidic fibroblast growth factors (FGFs) are closely related molecules that show a similar range of biological activities. They differ, however, in some of their physical and chemical properties and in their tissue distribution (Gospodarowicz et al. 1986).

Both basic FGF (bFGF) and acidic FGF (aFGF) are mitogenic in vitro for a wide range of cells primarily of mesodermal origin, although bFGF is considerably more potent than aFGF. These FGF-sensitive cell types include capillary endothelial cells, fibroblasts, vascular smooth-muscle cells, osteoblasts, and chondrocytes. In addition, FGFs have been shown to be chemotactic in vitro and to have neurotrophic activity. In vivo, they are angiogenic, as they have the ability to stimulate the proliferation of new capillaries in model systems such as the rabbit cornea and the chick chorioallantoic membrane. The biological relevance of FGFs has not yet been clearly established; however, bFGF in particular has been implicated in processes such as tissue repair and in the abnormal vascularization that supports the growth of solid tumors and causes diseases such as diabetic retinopathy.

bFGF has been purified from a variety of tissues, such as pituitary, brain, hypothalamus, retina, adrenal gland, corpus luteum, kidney, and placenta, and from several tumors and tumor cell lines. In contrast, aFGF has so far only been isolated from neural tissues such as brain, hypothalamus, and retina. The purification of FGFs has been greatly facilitated by the finding that they bind with a very high affinity to heparin-Sepharose (Shing et al. 1984). bFGF elutes from heparin-Sepharose columns at about 1.5–2.0 M NaCl, and aFGF elutes at about 1.1 M NaCl. Amino acid sequence analysis of the bovine FGFs (Esch et al. 1985a,b; Gimenez-Gallego et al. 1985) showed 55% homology between bFGF and aFGF.

Neither bFGF nor aFGF Has a Signal Peptide

We isolated a bFGF cDNA clone from a bovine pituitary library (Abraham et al. 1986b). Nucleotide sequence analysis revealed an open

24

reading frame of 155 codons, starting with a potential initiator methionine. This reading frame encoded the largest form of bFGF that had been sequenced (146 amino acids) plus an amino-terminal extension of nine codons. The sequence upstream of the proposed initiation codon was exceedingly G-C-rich and was thus unlikely to be a coding region. Further evidence supporting the conclusion that the primary translation product of bFGF contains 155 amino acids came from a comparison with the amino-terminal sequence of bovine aFGF, obtained by sequencing a genomic fragment (Abraham et al. 1986b). This comparison showed that aFGF likewise had an amino-terminal extension, in this case of 15 codons, making a primary translation product also of 155 amino acids. The amino-terminal extensions of the two factors are highly homologous, yet upstream the sequences in the proposed 5'-untranslated regions diverge completely.

Both bFGF and aFGF are growth factors that have been shown to interact with membrane-associated receptors. It would therefore be expected that FGFs are secreted proteins. However, examination of the amino-terminal sequences described above shows no sign of a conventional signal peptide. The mechanism by which FGFs leave the cell in which they are synthesized is currently unclear. Possibilities include release from the cell on lysis at the site of tissue damage, release by a specialized mechanism, and transport across the membrane in association with an extracellular matrix component such as heparan sulfate, to which FGFs are known to bind tightly.

bFGF mRNA Is Not Actively Synthesized in Tissues That Store bFGF Protein

The bovine bFGF cDNA clone was used as a hybridization probe to screen several human cDNA libraries (Abraham et al. 1986a). Clones were isolated at a very low level (average 1 in 500,000) and, in several cases, represented copies of unspliced transcripts. These cDNA cloning results, and the difficulties we have experienced in detecting bFGF mRNA in Northern blotting the RNAs that were used to make the libraries, are inconsistent with the quantities of bFGF protein that can be isolated from tissues. It would appear that the bFGF gene is normally not actively transcribed in these tissues and that the protein is stored. Such storage could be in an intracellular form or in an extracellular form associated with glycosaminoglycans such as heparan sulfate.

Human and Bovine bFGFs Are Highly Homologous Proteins

The nucleotide sequence of human bFGF was determined from several incomplete cDNA clones and from genomic clones (see below). A comparison of the encoded human amino acid sequence with that of

GTTGAGTC ACGGCTGGTT GCGCACGAAA AGCCCCGCAG TGTGGAGAAA GCCTAAACGT GGTTTGGGTG

GTCGCGGGGT TGGGCGGGGG TGACTTTTGG GGGATAAGGG GCGGTGGAGC CCAAAGCCCT GCCGCGGCCT CCGACGCGCG CTCGCCTCTC

CCCGCCCCCC GACTGAGGCC GGGCTCCCCG CCGGACTGAT GTCGCGCGCT TGCCGTGTTGT GGCCGAAGCC GCCGAACTCA GAGGCCGGCC CCAGAAAACC CGACCGAGTA

GGGGGCGGCG CGCAGGAGGG AGGAGAACTG GGGGCGCGGG AGGCTGGTGG GTGTGGGGGG TGGAGATGTA GAAGATGTGA CGCCCCGGCC CGGCGGGTGC CAGATTAGCG

GACCGGCTGCC CGCGGGTTGCA ACCGGATCCC GGGCGCTGCA GCTTGGGAGG CGGCTCTCCC CAGGCGGCGT CCGGCGGCGC GCGCGGAGAC ACCCATCTGT GAACCCCAGG TCCCGGGCCG

CCGGCTCGCC GCCCACCAGG GCCGGCGGGA CAGAAGAGCG GCCGAGCGGC TCGGAGGCTGG GGGACCGCGG GCGCTGCCGG GCGGGAGGCT GGGGGCCGG

GGCCGGGGCC GTGCCCGGAG CGGGTCGCGGAG CGGGCGGGGG GCCGGGCGGG ACGGCCGGCTC CCCGCCGCGGC TCCAGCGGCT CGGGGATCCC GGCCGGCCCC CGCAGGGACC

ATG GCA GCC GGG ATC ACC ACG CTG CCC GCC CTG CCC GAG GAT GGC GGC AGC GGC GGC TTG CCC CGC CAC GGC GCC TTC CCG CCC GGC CAC TTC AAG GAC CCC AAG
Met Ala Ala Gly Ser Ile Thr Thr Leu Pro Ala Leu Pro Glu Asp Gly Gly Ser Gly Gly Phe Pro Arg His Gly Ala Phe Pro Pro Gly His Phe Lys Asp Pro Lys
1   10   20   30

CGG CTG TAC TGC AAA AAC GGG GGC TTC TTC CTG CGC ATC CAC CCC GAC GGC CGA GTT GAC GGG GTC CGG GAG AAG AGC GAC CCT CAC A gt
Arg Leu Tyr Cys Lys Asn Gly Gly Phe Phe Leu Arg Ile His Pro Asp Gly Arg Val Asp Gly Val Arg Glu Lys Ser Asp Pro His I
40   50

gagtgcgaccgctctccgcctcatttcgtgggttctcg..............aaggctctttcctctgtgggtgctacaaagataattttttcccgtt

acag TC AAG CTA CAA CTT CAA GCA GAA GAG AGA GGA GTT GTG TCT ATC AAA GGA GTG TGT GCT AAC CGT TAC CTG GCT ATG AAG GAA GAT
     le Lys Leu Gln Leu Gln Ala Glu Glu Arg Gly Val Val Ser Ile Lys Gly Val Cys Ala Asn Arg Tyr Leu Ala Met Lys Glu Asp
     70   80

```
GGA AGA TTA CTG GCT TCT gtaagcatactttctgtttcacacgtttttgttagcttttattgctgt............taataataataatgataat
Gly Arg Leu Ala Ser
        90

aataacaggtaattcttccttattttcag AAA TGT GTT ACG GAT GAG TGT TTC TTT GAA CGA TTG GAA TCT AAT AAC TAC AAT ACT TAC CGG
                              Lys Cys Val Thr Asp Glu Cys Phe Phe Glu Arg Leu Glu Ser Asn Asn Tyr Asn Thr Tyr Arg
                                                    100                                     110

TCA AGG AAA TAC ACC AGT TGG TAT GTG GCA TTG AAA CGA ACT GGG CAG TAT AAA CTT GGA TCC AAA ACA GGA CCT GGG CAG AAA GCT ATA
Ser Arg Lys Tyr Thr Ser Trp Tyr Val Ala Leu Lys Arg Thr Gly Gln Tyr Lys Leu Gly Ser Lys Thr Gly Pro Gly Gln Lys Ala Ile
                    120                             130                                     140

CTT TTT CTT CCA ATG TCT GCT AAG AGC TGA TTTTAATGGC CACATCTAAT CTCATTTCAC ATGAAAGAAG AAGTATATTT TAGAAATTTG TTAATGAGAG TA
Leu Phe Leu Pro Met Ser Ala Lys Ser Ter
                150

AAGAAAA TAAATGTGTA TAGCTCAGTT TGGATAATTG GTCAAACAAT TTTTTATCCA GTAGTA
```

Figure 1 Partial nucleotide sequence of the human bFGF gene. The encoded amino acids are numbered 1–155, assuming that translation initiates with the methionine labeled 1. The first and last 50 bases of each intron are shown in lowercase letters. Possible binding sites for the transcription factor Sp1 in the 5′-flanking sequences are marked by a heavy underline. Possible translation initiation codons in this upstream region are marked by asterisks. The 5′ end of the longest cDNA clone is marked by an arrow. A potential polyadenylation signal in the 3′-untranslated region is boxed.

27

```
                                                   ***
TTGTTCAATT TCTTACAGTC TTGAAAGCGC CACAAGCAGC AGCTGCTGAG CC

ATG GCT GAA GGG GAA ATC ACC ACC TTC ACA GCC CTG ACC GAG AAG TTT AAT CTG CCT CCA GGG AAT TAC AAG CCC AAA CTC CTC TAC
MET Ala Glu Gly Glu Ile Thr Thr Phe Thr Ala Leu Thr Glu Lys Phe Asn Leu Pro Pro Gly Asn Tyr Lys Pro Lys Leu Leu Tyr
 1                          10                          20                          30

TGT AAC GGG GGC CAC TTC CTG AGG ATC CTT CGG GAT GGC ACA GTG GAT GGG ACA AGG GAC AGC GAC GAC CAG CAC A gtaagcccatctc
Cys Ser Asn Gly Gly His Phe Leu Arg Ile Leu Arg Asp Gly Thr Val Asp Gly Thr Arg Asp Ser Asp Gln His I
                    40                          50

tatggcaccccctttccctttctgacatcttctgtag.........agtgtttatttactttgctgtgttatttattccag TT CAG CTG CAG CTC AGT
                                                                                   le Gln Leu Gln Leu Ser
                                                                                             60

GCG GAA AGC GTG GGG GAG GTG TAT ATA AAG AGT ACC GAG ACT GGC CAG TAC TTG GCC ATG ACC GAC GGG CTT TTA TAC GGC TCA gta
Ala Glu Ser Val Gly Glu Val Tyr Ile Lys Ser Thr Glu Thr Gly Gln Tyr Leu Ala Met Thr Asp Gly Leu Leu Tyr Gly Ser
           70                          80                          90

agtatgaagtagacatgctccagacgttggcctggtt.........tgtgaaactactcactgattgtcctacctcttgtggtttatcttttag CAG ACA CCA
                                                                                                 Gln Thr Pro

AAT GAG GAA TGT TTC TTG CTG GAA AGG CTG GAG GAG AAC CAT TAC AAC ACC TAT ATA TCC AAG AAG CAT GCA GAG AAG AAT TGG TTT GTT
Asn Glu Glu Cys Phe Leu Leu Glu Arg Leu Glu Glu Asn His Tyr Asn Thr Tyr Ile Ser Lys Lys His Ala Glu Lys Asn Trp Phe Val
                    100                          110                          120

GGC CTC AAG AAG AAT GGG AGC TGC AAA CGC GGT CCT CGG ACT CAC TAT GGC CAG AAA GCA ATC TTG TTT CTC CCC CTG CCA GTC TCT TCT
Gly Leu Lys Lys Asn Gly Ser Cys Lys Arg Gly Pro Arg Thr His Tyr Gly Gln Lys Ala Ile Leu Phe Leu Pro Leu Pro Val Ser Ser
                    130                          140                          150

GAT TAA AGAGATCTGT TCTGGGTGTT GACCACTCCA GAGAAGTTTC GAGGGGTCCT CACCTGGTTG ACCCAAAAAT GTTCCCTTGA
Asp  .
```

Figure 2 Partial nucleotide sequence of the human aFGF gene. The encoded amino acids are numbered 1–155, assuming that translation initiates with the methionine labeled 1. An in-frame termination codon immediately upstream of the initiator methionine is marked with asterisks.

28

bovine bFGF showed that only 2 of the 155 amino acids differed. This level of homology, 98.7%, is exceptionally high, implying that bFGF has a highly conserved function and that there has been a strong selection pressure for maintenance of the sequence.

bFGF and aFGF Have Similar Gene Structures
We have isolated both bFGF (Abraham et al. 1986a) and aFGF (A. Mergia et al., in prep.) human genomic clones. Nucleotide sequences of the two genes are shown in Figures 1 and 2. The coding sequence for human aFGF agrees with that obtained by Jaye et al. (1986) for a human aFGF clone isolated from a brain stem cDNA library.

bFGF and aFGF have similar gene structures, with two introns located at identical positions. The two genes are large; in the case of bFGF, the minimum size of the gene is 34 kb. The gene for bFGF is on human chromosome 4, and that for aFGF is on human chromosome 5 (Mergia et al. 1986).

Heparin-binding Endothelial-cell Mitogens Are Encoded by Either the Single-copy bFGF or the Single-copy aFGF Gene
Human genomic Southern blot analysis showed that both bFGF and aFGF are encoded by single-copy genes; no related sequences were detected under conditions of low hybridization stringency. It would therefore appear that all of the cationic, endothelial-cell mitogens that have been described (pI 9.6, m.w. 14,000–18,000, elution from heparin-Sepharose at 1.5–2.0 M NaCl) are products of the single bFGF gene. Similarly, all of the anionic, endothelial-cell mitogens that have been described (pI 5.5, m.w. 14,000–18,000, elution from heparin-Sepharose at 1.1 M NaCl) are products of the single aFGF gene. In both cases, differences in molecular weights among the purified factors probably represent variations in amino-terminal proteolytic processing, possibly occurring during purification.

Capillary Endothelial Cells and Some Tumor Cell Lines Express the bFGF Gene
Northern blot analysis showed that cultured capillary endothelial cells isolated, for example, from bovine brain or adrenal cortex contain two bFGF transcripts of 7.0 kb and 3.7 kb (Schweigerer et al. 1987a). The presence of bFGF transcripts, and of the protein (Schweigerer et al. 1987a), in endothelial cells raises the possibility that bFGF can act as an autocrine or paracrine factor stimulating capillary endothelial-cell growth (angiogenesis) at the site of tissue damage.

Identically sized bFGF transcripts have also been observed in several human tumor cell lines, such as the SK-HEp-1 hepatoma (Abraham et al. 1986b), and in a rhabdomyosarcoma (Schweigerer et al. 1987b). The production of bFGF by a solid tumor, either directly from the tumor cells or indirectly by endothelial cells at the site of the malignancy, may be involved in the neovascularization that is required to support the growth of the tumor.

DISCUSSION

The data described in this summary, along with those of Jaye et al. (1986), represent the first characterization of the genes encoding endothelial-cell mitogens. The availability of cloned DNA sequences for bFGF and aFGF should help to provide answers to questions concerning the biosynthesis of these mitogens. In particular, we would like to understand (1) the significance of maintaining two separate yet closely related factors with similar activities and (2) the mechanisms involved in the release of these factors from the cells in which they are synthesized.

ACKNOWLEDGMENTS

We thank L. Tarrice for preparing the manuscript and M. Matsumara and E. Stoelting for the artwork. This work was supported by the Biotechnology Research Partners and by a Small Business Innovation Research grant from the National Institute for General Medical Sciences.

REFERENCES

Abraham, J.A., J.L. Whang, A. Tumolo, A. Mergia, J. Friedman, D. Gospodarowicz, and J.C. Fiddes. 1986a. Human basic fibroblast growth factor: Nucleotide sequence and genomic organization. *EMBO J.* 5: 2523.

Abraham, J.A., A. Mergia, J.L. Whang, A. Tumolo, J. Friedman, K.A. Hjerrild, D. Gospodarowicz, and J.C. Fiddes. 1986b. Nucleotide sequence of a bovine clone encoding the angiogenic protein, basic fibroblast growth factor. *Science* 233: 545.

Esch, F., N. Ueno, A. Baird, F. Hill, L. Denoroy, N. Ling, D. Gospodarowicz, and R. Guillemin. 1985a. Primary structure of bovine brain acidic fibroblast growth factor (FGF). *Biochem. Biophys. Res. Commun.* 133: 554.

Esch, F., A. Baird, N. Ling, N. Ueno, F. Hill, L. Denoroy, R. Klepper, D. Gospodarowicz, P. Bohlen, and R. Guillemin. 1985b. Primary structure of bovine pituitary basic fibroblast growth factor (FGF) and comparison with the amino-terminal sequence of bovine brain acidic FGF. *Proc. Natl. Acad. Sci.* 82: 6507.

Gimenez-Gallego, G., J. Rodkey, C. Bennett, M. Rios-Candelore, J. DiSalvo, and K. Thomas. 1985. Brain-derived acidic fibroblast growth factor: Complete amino acid sequence and homologies. *Science* 230: 1385.

Gospodarowicz, D., G. Neufeld, and L. Schweigerer. 1986. Fibroblast growth factors. *Mol. Cell. Endocrinol.* 46: 187.

Jaye, M., R. Howk, W. Burgess, G.A. Ricca, I.-M. Chui, M.W. Ravera, S.J. O'Brien, W.C. Modi, T. Maciag, and W.N. Drohan. 1986. Human endothelial cell growth factor: Cloning, nucleotide sequence, and chromosome localization. *Science* **233:** 541.

Mergia, A., R. Eddy, J.A. Abraham, J.C. Fiddes, and T.B. Shows. 1986. The genes for basic and acidic fibroblast growth factors are on different human chromosomes. *Biochem. Biophys. Res. Commun.* **138:** 644.

Schweigerer, L., G. Neufeld, J. Friedman, J.A. Abraham, J.C. Fiddes, and D. Gospodarowicz. 1987a. Capillary endothelial cells express basic fibroblast growth factor, a mitogen that promotes their own growth. *Nature* **325:** 257.

Schweigerer, L., G. Neufeld, A. Mergia, J.A. Abraham, J.C. Fiddes, and D. Gospodarowicz. 1987b. Basic fibroblast growth factor in human rhabdomyosarcoma cells: Implications for the proliferation and neovascularization of myoblast-derived tumors. *Proc. Natl. Acad. Sci.* **84:** 842.

Shing, Y., J. Folkman, R. Sullivan, C. Butterfield, J. Murray, and M. Klagsbrun. 1984. Heparin affinity: Purification of a tumor-derived capillary endothelial cell growth factor. *Science* **223:** 1296.

31

Primary Structure of a Human Basic Fibroblast Growth Factor Derived from Protein and cDNA Sequencing

A. Sommer, M.T. Brewer, R.C. Thompson, D. Moscatelli,* M. Presta,*† and D.B. Rifkin*

Synergen, Inc., Boulder, Colorado 80301
*Department of Cell Biology and Kaplan Center
New York University Medical Center, New York, New York 10016

We have isolated from term placenta a protein that induces the production of the proteases plasminogen activator and collagenase in bovine capillary cells (Moscatelli et al. 1986). In addition, this protein is a potent chemotactic and mitogenic factor for these same cells (Moscatelli et al. 1986). These three activities have been postulated to be part of the angiogenic response (Gross et al. 1983) and may represent the in vitro equivalents of the dissolution of the basement membrane, the migration of endothelial cells, and the increased proliferation of cells seen during the growth of a new blood vessel. The isolated human placental protein has been shown to be angiogenic on the chick chorioallantoic membrane (Moscatelli et al. 1986). We have also characterized a protein from the human hepatoma cell line SK-HEp-1, which has similar biological and chemical characteristics and which cross-reacts with antibodies prepared against the placental protein (Presta et al. 1986).

We have determined the amino acid sequence of the angiogenesis factor from placenta. It appears to be a human basic fibroblast growth factor (bFGF), since it is highly homologous to bovine pituitary bFGF (Esch et al. 1985). The complete sequence is derived from a combination of protein sequencing of the placental protein and nucleotide sequencing of a cDNA clone from SK-HEp-1, which codes for a protein identical to the placental protein. The human placental protein sequence indicates, however, that translation of the corresponding mRNA must initiate 5′ to the start site proposed for other bFGFs (Abraham et al. 1986a,b).

---

†Present address: Institute of General Pathology, Faculty of Medicine, University of Brescia, Italy.

Protein Sequence of Human Placental Angiogenesis Factor

Peptides of the human placental angiogenesis factor (hPAF) to be used for protein sequencing were generated by digestion of the purified native placental protein with endoproteinase Lys-C, submaxillaris protease, and staphylococcal protease V8. Peptides were reduced and carboxymethylated, separated by reversed-phase high-performance liquid chromatography, and sequenced by automated Edman degradation.

The primary structure of the human placental protein is shown in Figure 1. The amino-terminal amino acid sequence was established by automated Edman degradation of purified, uncleaved placental protein and confirmed by the sequence of a peptide isolated from the endoproteinase Lys-C digest. The yield of phenylthiohydantoin amino acids obtained upon sequencing of the uncleaved protein was, however, 20–40% of that normally expected. Thus, a substantial portion of the placental protein may be blocked at the amino terminus. Identification

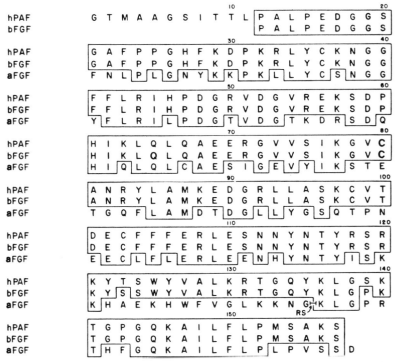

Figure 1 Primary structure and protein sequence homology among hPAF, bovine bFGF (Esch et al. 1985), and bovine aFGF (Gimenez-Gallego et al. 1985). Identical amino acid residues at a given position are enclosed in boxes.

of the carboxy-terminal residue as serine is based on (1) sequence analysis of a Lys-C peptide that terminated with the sequence ----S-A-K-S and (2) cDNA sequence data (Fig. 2) that reveal a terminator codon immediately following DNA coding for the sequence ----S-A-K-S. Residues 18–21, 30–33, 117–120, and 131–135 were not unambiguously identified by protein sequencing and were deduced from the cDNA sequence (Fig. 2).

SK-HEp-1 cDNA Sequence

SK-HEp-1 cells have been shown to synthesize a protein that cross-reacts with antibodies prepared against the placental protein (Presta et al. 1986). These cells were used as a source of mRNA for construction of a cDNA library in λgt10.

Two oligonucleotide probes, a 192-fold degenerate 17-mer corresponding to the placental protein amino acid sequence I-K-G-V-C-A (Fig. 1, residues 76–81) and a 256-fold degenerate 20-mer corresponding to the amino acid sequence Y-C-K-N-G-G-F (Fig. 1 residues 35–41) were synthesized and used to screen approximately 1.2×10^6 plaques. Five plaques were found to hybridize to both probes, and one of these was selected for DNA sequencing. A partial sequence of this cDNA is shown in Figure 2. The sequence contains an open reading frame for an amino acid sequence, which is completely in agreement with the primary structure of the placental protein.

DISCUSSION

We have determined the primary structure of hPAF by a combination of protein sequencing and cDNA sequencing. Inspection of the primary structure (Fig. 1) reveals the presence of 157 amino acids with a calculated molecular weight of 17,464. A comparison of the primary structure of the hPAF with that of bovine pituitary bFGF and bovine brain aFGF is shown in Figure 1. It is evident that (1) the hPAF is a member of the bFGF family, (2) there is an 11-amino-acid extension at the amino terminus of the placental protein that is not present in the bovine bFGF isolated by Esch et al. (1985), (3) there are two amino acid substitutions (residues 123 and 139) relative to bovine bFGF, and (4) there exists a substantial homology between hPAF and bovine aFGF.

The structures of cDNA clones encoding bovine bFGF and human bFGF have recently been reported by Abraham et al. (1986a,b), who have presented arguments that a methionine homologous to Met-3 of the human placental bFGF (see Figs. 1 and 2) is the translational initiation site. Our protein sequence of the placental bFGF indicates unequivocally that this methionine cannot be the only translational start

Figure 2 — Nucleotide sequence and predicted translation of the hPAF cDNA clone (open reading frame). Reading left to right (N-terminus → C-terminus); numbers above codons are nucleotide positions.

nt	codons / amino acids
1–60	GGG ACC ATG GCA GCC GGG AGC ATC ACC ACG **(30)** CTG CCC GCC TTG CCC GAG GAT GGC GGC AGC **(60)**
	Gly Thr Met Ala Ala Gly Ser Ile Thr Thr · Leu Pro Ala Leu Pro Glu Asp Gly Gly Ser
61–120	GGC GCC TTC CCG CCC GGC CAC TTC AAG GAC **(90)** CCC CGG TAC CTG CTG TGC AAA AAC GGG GGC **(120)**
	Gly Ala Phe Pro Pro Gly His Phe Lys Asp · Pro Arg Tyr Leu Leu Cys Lys Asn Gly Gly
121–180	TTC CTG CGC ATC ATC CAC CAC ATC GAC CGA **(150)** GTT GGG GTC GTG TCT TCT GTG AGC GAC CCT **(180)**
	Phe Leu Arg Ile Ile His His Ile Asp Arg · Val Gly Val Val Ser Ser Val Ser Asp Pro
181–240	CAC ATC AAG CTA CAA CAA ATG AAG AGA GGA **(210)** GAG GCA GAA GCA GTG CTG AAA GGA GTG TGT **(240)**
	His Ile Lys Leu Gln Gln Met Lys Arg Gly · Glu Ala Glu Ala Val Leu Lys Gly Val Cys
241–300	GCT AAC CGT TAC CTG ATG GCT AAT AAC TCT **(270)** GAA TTG TAC AAT GTC TAC CGC TCA GTT ACG **(300)**
	Ala Asn Arg Tyr Leu Met Ala Asn Asn Ser · Glu Leu Tyr Asn Val Tyr Arg Ser Val Thr
301–360	GAT GAG TGT TTC TTT TTT GAA TCT TTG GAT **(330)** GAA GCA GTG GCA TAC TAC CGC TGT TCA AGG **(360)**
	Asp Glu Cys Phe Phe Phe Glu Ser Leu Asp · Glu Ala Val Ala Tyr Tyr Arg Cys Ser Arg
361–420	AAA TAC ACC AGT TGG TAT CAG ACT AAA CGA **(390)** AAA ACT AAT TAC TCT TAC CGC TCC TCA AAA **(420)**
	Lys Tyr Thr Ser Trp Tyr Gln Thr Lys Arg · Lys Thr Asn Tyr Ser Tyr Arg Ser Ser Lys
421–468	ACA GGA CCT GGG CAG AAA GCT ATA CTT TTT **(450)** CTT CCA ATG TCT GCT TCT AAG AGC AGC TGA
	Thr Gly Pro Gly Gln Lys Ala Ile Leu Phe · Leu Pro Met Ser Ala Ser Lys Ser Ser End

Figure 2 Nucleotide sequence of a cDNA clone derived from human hepatoma mRNA (SK-HEp-1 cell line). The predicted translation product of the open reading frame is also shown and is completely in agreement with the primary structure of the hPAF as established by protein sequencing.

35

site. A clear definition of the initial translation product of human placental bFGF mRNA will require the isolation of appropriate cDNA clones, which is presently under way in our laboratory.

ACKNOWLEDGMENTS

We thank Ms. Julie A. Wilson and Mr. R. Manejias for their excellent technical assistance. This work was supported in part by grants from the National Institutes of Health and the American Cancer Society to D.B.R. D.M. was supported by an investigatorship from the New York Heart Association. M.P. was supported by a fellowship from the Juvenile Diabetes Foundation International.

REFERENCES

Abraham, J.A., J.L. Whang, A. Tumolo, A. Mergia, J. Friedman, D. Gospodarowicz, and J.C. Fiddes. 1986a. Human basic fibroblast growth factor: Nucleotide sequence and genomic organization. *EMBO J.* 5: 2523.

Abraham, J.A., A. Mergia, J.L. Whang, A. Tumolo, J. Friedman, K.A. Hjerrild, D. Gospodarowicz, and J.C. Fiddes. 1986b. Nucleotide sequence of a bovine clone encoding the angiogenic protein, basic fibroblast growth factor. *Science* 233: 545.

Esch, F., A. Baird, N. Ling, N. Ueno, F. Hill, L. Denoroy, R. Klepper, D. Gospodarowicz, P. Bohlen, and R. Guillemin. 1985. Primary structure of bovine pituitary basic fibroblast growth factor (FGF) and comparison with the amino-terminal sequence of bovine brain acidic FGF. *Proc. Natl. Acad. Sci.* 82: 6507.

Gimenez-Gallego, G., J. Rodkey, C. Bennett, M. Rios-Candelore, J. DiSalvo, and K. Thomas. 1985. Brain-derived acidic fibroblast growth factor: Complete amino acid sequence and homologies. *Science* 230: 1385.

Gross, J.L., D. Moscatelli, and D.B. Rifkin. 1983. Increased capillary endothelial cell protease activity in response to angiogenic stimuli *in vitro*. *Proc. Natl. Acad. Sci.* 80: 2623.

Moscatelli, D., M. Presta, and D.B. Rifkin. 1986. Purification of a factor from human placenta that stimulates capillary endothelial cell protease production, DNA synthesis, and migration. *Proc. Natl. Acad. Sci.* 83: 2091.

Presta, M., D. Moscatelli, J. Joseph-Silverstein, and D.B. Rifkin. 1986. Purification from a human hepatoma cell line of a basic fibroblast growth factor-like molecule that stimulates capillary endothelial cell plasminogen activator production, DNA synthesis, and migration. *Mol. Cell. Biol.* 6: 4060.

Modulation of Eye-derived Growth Factor Activity and Fixation in the Eye

Y. Courtois

Unite de Recherches Gerontologiques
INSERM U. 118, CNRS UA 630 75016 Paris, France

Study of the control of growth and differentiation of the embryonic or adult lens has demonstrated that adult bovine retina contains a potent growth factor, which was isolated through its ability to stimulate lens epithelial cell proliferation in vitro (Arruti and Courtois 1978). The presence of similar mitogenic activity in other eye tissues, such as iris or vitreous, was also demonstrated. Because of its ubiquitous distribution, we named it eye-derived growth factor (EDGF) (Barritault et al. 1981). We also demonstrated that this growth factor, while still not fully purified, was able to stimulate many cell types, as this was the case for the bovine brain-derived growth factor (BDGF) purified with the same technology.

EDGF, like BDGF and fibroblast growth factor (FGF), was able to stimulate various cell types in vitro, including bovine aortic endothelial cells. Furthermore, experiments showed that EDGF was angiogenic, since when delivered at a very slow rate by an osmotic pump within the rabbit corneal stroma, it induced the proliferation of capillaries from the limbus (Thompson et al. 1982). Thus, it seemed that EDGF might play several roles in eye physiology or pathology. It might be a ubiquitous signal that, by a paracrine route, controls either lens development or regeneration, corneal wound healing, or neovascular induction in retina. It is on this latter putative pathological role that several groups have isolated growth factors such as retina-derived growth factor (RDGF) (D'Amore et al. 1984). Pituitary FGF also displayed high angiogenic activity.

Recent advances in purification, achieved mainly through chromatography of the various extracts on heparin-Sepharose, have allowed complete purification of these growth factors and have shown that they belong to two families of fibroblast growth factors, acidic FGF (aFGF) and basic FGF (bFGF), analogous to EDGF II and EDGF I, respectively (for review, see Gospodarowicz et al. 1986). These major advances have raised several questions related to the paracrine and autocrine roles of these growth factors: (1) Where are they synthesized and stored within the retina? (2) Do they have an autocrine role in normal physiology? (3) How are they transported out to reach other target tissues of the eye, and what determines their affinity for these tissues? (4) What are the cofactors that could modulate their activity? Do the acidic and basic forms have similar roles? (5) What are the various normal or pathological situations in which their angiogenic activity is released in the retina?

The first question concerns the synthesis and storage of EDGF in the different layers of the retina. Although the site of synthesis is still not known, recent experiments (Pettman et al. 1986) have demonstrated by immunocytochemistry that an astroglial growth factor (AGF) analogous to FGF can be localized in all rat brain neurons. We have used poly- and monoclonal antibodies against AGF and have observed a specific staining of several layers of adult bovine retina. The disk area was the most intensely labeled in the photoreceptors, followed by the area containing the bipolar cells and the ganglion cells. The localization of EDGF in the photoreceptor was confirmed by a recent investigation in which we determined EDGF mitogenic activity of isolated rod outer segments on bovine retinal pigmented epithelial cells or lens epithelial cells (Plouet et al. 1986).

EDGF mitogenic activity was determined on bovine lens epithelial cells and on retinal pigmented cells (Table 1). S-antigen is a soluble 48K protein involved in phototransduction and present only in the photoreceptors. In these experiments, only the activity of the soluble fractions was reported. This allowed us to monitor the degree of contamination of the various layers by photoreceptor proteins during rod outer segment membrane preparation. We have found EDGF activity in both soluble and insoluble membranes with a distribution of 1 : 2, respectively (Plouet et al. 1986). It was then tempting to assess the role of EDGF in phototransduction. We analyzed EDGF affinity for rod outer segment membrane proteins and showed that EDGF can be partially released from extensively washed membranes at low ionic strength in a light-dependent manner. In addition, EDGF is readily released by ATP but not by GTP. These results suggest that EDGF plays an autocrine role in the photoreceptor physiology, probably in phototransduction.

The paracrine role of EDGF implies that it diffuses from its source to the target tissue. Since our data indicated that it could modulate protein synthesis in lens organ culture, we also looked for EDGF-binding sites in the eye. In a series of experiments performed with iodinated aFGF and bFGF or EDGF I and II, we incubated fixed or unfixed frozen sections of the mouse embryonic eye with the growth factor and

Table 1 Distribution of EDGF and S-antigen in Various Layers of the Retina

Location	Dark-adapted retinas[a]		Light-adapted retinas	
	EDGF mitogenic activity (SU/retina)	S-antigen (μg/retina)	EDGF mitogenic activity (SU/retina)	S-antigen (μg/retina)
Inner layers	700	500	600	750
Rod cytosol	800	290	1150	290
Rod outer segment	90	70	120	100
Interphotoreceptor matrix	560	75	400	15
Rod outer segment of interphotoreceptor matrix	10	8	18	105

[a] SU = Standard unit of activity.

39

revealed their localization by autoradiography (Fig. 1). Our recent data (Jeanny et al. 1987) demonstrate that EDGF I and II bind specifically to all basement membranes of the eye, including blood vessel basement membrane. The binding can only be displaced with an excess of growth factor or by treating the sections with heparitinase. EDGF I has more affinity than EDGF II, probably reflecting the higher isoelectric point of the former.

It is thus tempting to propose that the basement membrane–growth factor interaction has a significant meaning in controlling the movement and the activity of these growth factors during development and pathology. The nature of this interaction is probably related to the high affinity of EDGFs and FGFs for heparin. Heparin and a synthetic pentasaccharide can both stimulate the mitogenic activity of EDGF II (aFGF) (Uhlrich et al. 1986). Further experiments performed with retinal extracts and purified growth factors indicate that the heparin effect (stimulation or inhibition) on EDGF mitogenic activity in vitro can produce exactly opposite effects in the presence or absence of fetal calf serum. These results suggest that the binding of the growth factors to the basement membrane is mediated through a heparin-like compo-

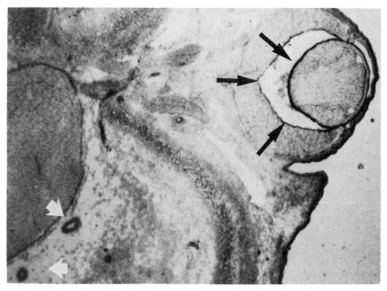

Figure 1 Fixation of iodinated bFGF on a frozen section of mouse 15-day embryonic eye basement membrane. Note that all basement membranes are outlined, to different extents, by the fixation of iodinated FGF. White arrows indicate heavy labeling in cross sections of the main arteries near the neural tube. Black arrows indicate labeling in eye basement membrane.

nent or an associated protein that can positively or negatively regulate the paracrine mitogenic activity of EDGF. The different behaviors of EDGF I and EDGF II may also influence their sequestration in the extracellular matrix and their ability to diffuse out.

The experiments reported here tend to demonstrate that, although their respective roles are not yet elucidated, EDGF I and II may play a central role in the normal physiology of the retina, perhaps as a pacemaker with multiple functions in the eye. The angiogenic activity found in adult retinal extracts may thus be released consecutively, resulting in disruption of the normal organization of photoreceptors or other neural cells by injuries or pathological conditions (as in RCS rats) or in macular degeneration.

ACKNOWLEDGMENTS

I thank all of my collaborators and colleagues from other laboratories who participated at some stage of this work, and particularly C. Arruti, D. Barritault, J. Courty, M.F. Counis, J.C. Jeanny, J. Plouet, D. Raulais, J. Tassin, M. Vigny, O. Lagente, M. Lenfant, N. Fayein, S. Uhlrich, M. Diry, J.P. Faure, M. Laurent, B. Chevallier, and F. Mascarelli.

REFERENCES

Arruti, C. and Y. Courtois. 1978. Morphological changes and growth stimulation of bovine epithelial lens cells by a retinal extract in vitro. *Exp. Cell. Res.* **117**: 283.

Barritault, D., C. Arruti, and Y. Courtois. 1981. Is there an ubiquitous growth factor in the eye? Proliferation induced in different cell types by eye derived growth factor. *Differentiation* **18**: 29.

D'Amore, P.A., B.M. Glaser, S.K. Brunson, and A. Fenselou. 1984. Angiogenic activity from bovine retina: Partial purification and characterization. *Proc. Natl. Acad. Sci.* **78**: 3068.

Gospodarowicz, D., G. Neufeld, and L. Schweigerer. 1986. Molecular and biological characterization of fibroblast growth factor, an angiogenic factor which also controls the proliferation of mesoderm and neuroectoderm derived cells. *Cell. Differ.* **19**: 1.

Jeanny, J.C., N. Fayein, M. Moenner, B. Chevallier, D. Barritault, and Y. Courtois. 1987. Specific fixation of bovine brain and retinal acidic and basic fibroblasts growth factors to mouse embryonic eye basement membranes. *Exp. Cell. Res.* (in press).

Pettman, B., G. Labourdette, M. Weibel, and M. Sensenbrenner. 1986. The brain fibroblast growth factor (FGF) is localised in neurons. *Neurosci. Lett.* **68**: 125.

Plouet, J., F. Mascarelli, O. Lagente, C. Dorey, G. Lorans, J.P. Faure, and Y. Courtois. 1986. Eye derived growth factor: A component of rod outer segment implicated in phototransduction: Retinal signal systems, degeneration and transplant (ed. E. Agardh and B. Ehinger), p. 311. Elsevier Science.

Thompson, P., C. Arruti, D. Maurice, J. Plouet, D. Barritault, and Y. Courtois. 1982. Angiogenic activity of a cell growth regulating factor derived from the retina. In *Problem of normal and genetically abnormal retina* (ed. R. Clayton), p. 63. Academic Press, New York.

Uhlrich, S., O. Lagente, M. Lenfant, and Y. Courtois. 1986. Effect of heparin on the stimulation of nonvascular cells by human acidic and basic FGF. *Biochem. Biophys. Res. Commun.* **137**: 1205.

A Heparin Hexasaccharide Fragment Able to Bind to Anionic Endothelial Cell Growth Factor: Preparation and Structure

J.C. Lormeau, M. Petitou, J. Choay, and B. Perly*

Institut Choay, 75782 Paris Cedex 16, France
*CEA, IRDI/DPC, 91191 Gif-sur-Yvette, Cedex, France

Among growth factors, those classified as fibroblast growth factors (FGFs) and endothelial cell growth factors (ECGFs) have a strong affinity for heparin. The technique of affinity chromatography on matrix-linked heparin has greatly improved their purification process and is now widely used (Lobb et al. 1986).

It has been suggested that heparin could be involved in the modulation of growth factor activity, thus indirectly participating in the control of cell growth (Schreiber et al. 1985). In addition, it was shown that heparin and its fragments, either alone or in combination with steroids, play a role in the process of angiogenesis (Folkman et al. 1983).

The heterogeneity of heparin preparations with regard to their molecular weight and structure is now well documented (Casu 1985); however, it is not known which structural features are involved in the binding of heparin to growth factors. The present studies were undertaken as a contribution to the settlement of this point. To this end, commercial heparin was degraded into fragments, which were fractionated by gel filtration followed by affinity chromatography on an acidic FGF (aFGF) matrix and then studied by physicochemical methods (nuclear magnetic resonance [NMR] and high-performance liquid chromatography [HPLC]).

Preparation of Heparin Fragments Homogeneous in Size

A commercial preparation of pig mucosal heparin was cleaved by nitrous acid under controlled conditions. The resulting oligosaccharides were reduced with sodium borohydride and then fractionated on a column of Ultrogel AcA 202 into fragments ranging from disaccharides to tetradecasaccharides. These compounds were analyzed by

43

gel permeation HPLC and were proved to be homogeneous in size. In contrast, analysis of these fragments by ion-exchange HPLC revealed that, despite their size homogeneity, they were a complex mixture of variously charged species (Fig. 1).

Affinity Chromatography

An aFGF-Sepharose matrix, consisting of aFGF covalently linked to Sepharose, was prepared using bovine brain aFGF and packed into a column. An overloading amount of tetra-, hexa-, octa-, and decasaccharides was applied to the column, and, after extensive washing, bound oligosaccharides were eluted by increasing the ionic strength. Under our experimental conditions, a hexasaccharide was the shortest fragment retained on the column. This hexasaccharide was found to be practically homogeneous by ion-exchange HPLC (Fig. 1).

Determination of the Structure

The above hexasaccharide was analyzed by ^{13}C- and ^{1}H-NMR spectroscopy. Using bidimensional techniques of multiple-relay-correlation and nuclear-Overhauser-effect spectroscopy, the structure was proved to correspond to the hexasaccharide of Figure 2. This structure was confirmed by chemical degradation followed by analysis of the resulting

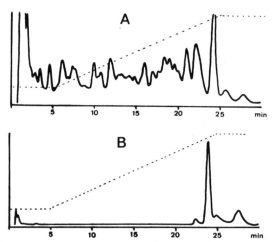

Figure 1 HPLC analysis of the mixture of hexasaccharides obtained from heparin after deaminative cleavage and gel filtration (A) and of the practically homogeneous hexasaccharide selected by aFGF-Sepharose affinity chromatography (B). A Pharmacia Mono Q HR 5/5 column (0.5 × 5 cm) was eluted at a flow rate of 1 ml/min with a gradient (0.5 → 1.5 M sodium chloride). UV detection (214 nm) was used to monitor the effluent.

44

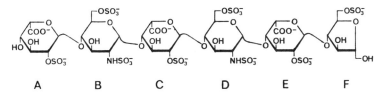

Figure 2 Structure of the hexasaccharide retained on the affinity column. (A,C,E) 2-O-sulfo-α-L-iduronic acid; (B,D) 6-O-sulfo-N-sulfo-α-D-glucosamine; (F) 6-O-sulfo-2,5-anhydro-D-mannitol.

fragments by HPLC and NMR. The hexasaccharide (Fig. 2) is derived from a sequence contained in the starting heparin and in which unit F is an N-sulfated glucosamine residue. Such a sequence is a trimer of 2-O-sulfo-α-L-iduronic acid $1 \rightarrow 4$ 6-O-sulfo-N-sulfo-α-D-glucosamine (Fig. 2, AB and CD), which is the most widespread disaccharide sequence in heparin.

DISCUSSION

Our results indicate that the minimal structure able to bind to Sepharose-linked aFGF is contained in hexasaccharide A-F (Fig. 2). Owing to the deaminative cleavage method used for splitting heparin, the reducing-end unit (F) of this hexasaccharide is a 2,5-anhydromannitol residue, derived from a glucosamine unit. Moreover, this method only leads to tetrasaccharides and hexasaccharides having such modified reducing-end units and cannot afford either an intact tetrasaccharide like A-D or a pentasaccharide like A-E. Therefore, one cannot exclude the possibility that such intact tetrasaccharide or pentasaccharide would bind to aFGF under our experimental conditions. These points are currently under investigation in our laboratory.

We are aware that the conformation of aFGF may be altered by covalent binding to the Sepharose matrix. Nevertheless, the hexasaccharide that we have characterized most likely represents a sequence in heparin able to accommodate aFGF. On the other hand, the milligram quantities of product required to conduct structural studies were, in a first approach, conveniently obtained through this simple process.

These first results show that a so-called regular heparin structure is able to bind to aFGF. This structure is widely distributed in heparin. It represents a high-charge-density domain of the heparin molecule and the question thus arises whether the binding of heparin to aFGF requires a specific sequence of monosaccharide residues, a high charge density, or both. This hexasaccharide sequence may also be viewed as an irregular sequence in heparan sulfate, where its true role might be to recognize growth factors.

ACKNOWLEDGMENT

The scientific assistance of Ms. G. Babinet is gratefully acknowledged.

REFERENCES

Casu, B. 1985. Structure and biological activity of heparin. *Adv. Carbohydr. Chem. Biochem.* **43**: 51.

Folkman, J., R. Langer, R.J. Linhardt, C. Haudenschild, and S. Taylor. 1983. Angiogenesis inhibition and tumor regression caused by heparin or a heparin fragment in the presence of cortisone. *Science* **221**: 719.

Lobb, R., J. Sasse, R. Sullivan, Y. Shing, P. D'Amore, J. Jacobs, and M. Klagsbrun. 1986. Purification and characterization of heparin-binding endothelial cell growth factors. *J. Biol. Chem.* **261**: 1924.

Schreiber, A.B., J. Kenney, W.J. Kowalski, R. Friesel, T. Mehlman, and T. Maciag. 1985. Interaction of endothelial cell growth factor with heparin: Characterization by receptor antibody recognition. *Proc. Natl. Acad. Sci.* **82**: 6138.

Presence of Basic Fibroblast Growth Factor in a Variety of Cells and Its Binding to Cells

D. Moscatelli, M. Presta,* J. Joseph-Silverstein, and D.B. Rifkin

Department of Cell Biology and Kaplan Cancer Center
New York University Medical Center, New York, New York 10016

During tumor angiogenesis, angiogenic factors released by the tumors stimulate endothelial cells of the neighboring capillaries to penetrate into the surrounding tissue, to migrate toward the source of the angiogenic factor, and to multiply, thereby forming a new network of capillaries supplying nutrients to the tissue. It is thought that these responses are correlated to three in vitro responses of capillary endothelial cells to angiogenic factors (Gross et al. 1983): stimulation of the production of the proteases plasminogen activator and collagenase, increased chemotaxis, and elevated rate of proliferation. We have used one of these responses, the increased production of plasminogen activator (PA) and collagenase by cultured bovine capillary endothelial (BCE) cells, as an assay for the purification of an angiogenic factor from term human placenta (Moscatelli et al. 1986a). The purified molecule was shown to have all three of the above properties proposed for an angiogenic factor (Moscatelli et al. 1986a). The purified molecule was identified as basic fibroblast growth factor (bFGF) on the basis of its similar chemical properties and a 98% amino acid sequence homology with bovine pituitary bFGF (Sommer et al., this volume).

Presence of bFGF-like Molecules in a Variety of Cells

In the purification of human bFGF from placenta, it was observed that all of the PA-stimulatory activity in the crude extracts copurified with bFGF, suggesting that the ability to stimulate PA production in BCE cells could be used as a rapid, quantitative assay for the presence of bFGF in tissues and cell extracts. Preliminary investigations showed that extracts of several cell lines were able to stimulate production of PA and collagenase in BCE cells in the same manner as the purified human bFGF, suggesting that bFGF-like molecules may be made by a wide

*Present address: Institute of General Pathology, University of Brescia, Brescia, Italy.

variety of cells. To investigate this possibility, extracts from ten different cell lines or strains were assayed for their ability to stimulate PA production in BCE cells.

Eight of the ten cell extracts tested contained PA-stimulatory activity. PA-stimulatory activity was present in human hepatoma, cervical carcinoma, histiocytic leukemia, and melanoma cells; human, chicken, and bovine embryonic fibroblasts; and bovine capillary endothelial cells (Moscatelli et al. 1986b). The amount of activity present in these cells had no relation to whether they were derived from normal or tumor tissue. To confirm that the PA-stimulatory activity was due to bFGF-like molecules, the extracts were subjected to heparin-Sepharose chromatography. Like bFGF, all of the PA-stimulatory activity bound to heparin-Sepharose and eluted with 2 M NaCl. No PA-stimulatory activity was eluted with a 0.5 M or a 1 M NaCl wash prior to the 2 M NaCl elution. As a further confirmation that the PA-stimulatory activity was due to bFGF-like molecules, we found that antibodies raised against the human placental bFGF would neutralize the PA-stimulatory activity of these extracts. These experiments demonstrate that a variety of cells, from both tumor and normal tissues, are able to synthesize bFGF-like molecules.

Basic FGF-like Molecules Remain Cell-associated

In the above experiments, PA-stimulatory activity was found only in cell extracts, not in the medium from the cell cultures. For several of the cell lines, we attempted to concentrate any bFGF-like molecules from the medium by heparin-Sepharose chromatography. Large quantities of medium that had been incubated on cells for 48 hours were passed over a heparin-Sepharose column, and the column was eluted with 2 M NaCl. No PA-stimulatory activity was detected in these experiments (Moscatelli et al. 1986b). These results suggested either that the bFGF-like molecules were not released into the medium or that any bFGF-like molecules that were released were rapidly inactivated.

To distinguish between these possibilities, human hepatoma cells were labeled with [^{35}S]methionine for 24 hours, and the medium and cell extracts from these cultures were incubated with antibodies against the human placental bFGF. A labeled bFGF-like molecule was immunoprecipitated from the cell extract, but not from the medium (Presta et al. 1986). This demonstrates that the bFGF-like molecules synthesized by these cells remain cell-associated.

Cell Binding Sites for bFGF

The purified human placental bFGF was labeled with ^{125}I, and the labeled molecule was shown to retain full biological activity. This

[125]I-labeled bFGF was used to investigate the presence of binding sites for bFGF on cells. For initial experiments, BHK cells were used, since they had been shown earlier to have receptors for bFGF (Neufeld and Gospodarowicz 1985). In contrast to the earlier study of BHK cells which had reported the presence of only high-affinity binding sites (Neufeld and Gospodarowicz 1985), our data indicated the presence of two binding sites for bFGF. The high-affinity binding had a dissociation constant of 2×10^{-11} M and had 80,000 sites per cell, and the low-affinity binding had a dissociation constant of 2×10^{-9} M and had 600,000 sites per cell. Binding to the high-affinity site was pH-sensitive, suggesting that this site represented the receptor. Binding to the low-affinity site was not affected by pH values down to 4.0.

Binding of ^{125}I-labeled bFGF to cells was not competed by a variety of other proteins, showing that the binding was specific. However, part of the binding could be competed with a heparin-binding protein that copurified with bFGF on heparin-Sepharose and did not cross-react with antibodies to the human placental bFGF. This suggested that the low-affinity binding might be due to binding to heparin-like molecules synthesized by the cells.

Since bFGF can be eluted from heparin-Sepharose with 2 M NaCl, we attempted to elute the ^{125}I-labeled bFGF from the cell with 2 M NaCl. When cells that had bound ^{125}I-labeled bFGF were washed with 2 M NaCl, a portion of the ^{125}I-labeled bFGF was released. Subsequent extraction of the cells with 0.5% Triton X-100 released the remaining ^{125}I-labeled bFGF. By Scatchard analysis, it was determined that the radioactivity released by the 2 M NaCl wash represented binding to the low-affinity sites, whereas the radioactivity released by the subsequent extraction represented binding to the high-affinity sites. Thus, by first washing cells that have bound ^{125}I-labeled bFGF with 2 M NaCl and then extracting with 0.5% Triton X-100, effects on low-affinity binding could be distinguished from effects on high-affinity binding.

Using these procedures, we found that heparin would compete strongly with ^{125}I-labeled bFGF binding to low-affinity sites, but not with binding to high-affinity sites. Heparan sulfate competed for binding to low-affinity sites at about 30-fold higher concentrations than heparin. Chondroitin sulfate, dermatan sulfate, and keratan sulfate had no effect on either low-affinity or high-affinity binding. These results suggested that the low-affinity binding represented binding to cell-associated heparin-like molecules. This conclusion was supported by the finding that by treating cells with heparinase, over 60% of the low-affinity binding was abolished with little effect on high-affinity binding. Together, all of these results support the interpretation that the high-affinity binding represents binding to cellular receptors for bFGF and the low-affinity binding represents binding to cell-associated heparin-like molecules.

A survey of a variety of other cultured cells showed that both high-affinity and low-affinity binding sites for bFGF are present on many cell types, including fibroblasts, sarcoma cells, melanoma cells, and capillary endothelial cells. To determine whether the binding to low-affinity sites played any role in the biological response of BCE cells to bFGF, BCE cells were incubated with human placental bFGF in the presence of heparin concentrations that competed completely for ^{125}I-labeled bFGF binding to low-affinity sites. In these cells, PA production was stimulated to the same extent as in cells incubated with human placental bFGF in the absence of heparin. These findings indicated that binding to the low-affinity site has no direct role in the stimulation of PA production in BCE cells. The low-affinity binding sites may act merely as a reservoir of bFGF around the cell.

DISCUSSION
These findings demonstrate that a variety of cells, from both normal and tumor tissues, contain bFGF-like molecules, suggesting that angiogenesis can be induced by injury to many types of cells. In normal cultures, most of the bFGF remains cell-associated. This may represent intracellular, nonsecreted bFGF. However, since a wide variety of cell types have low-affinity binding sites for bFGF, part of the cell-associated bFGF may be secreted bFGF that has bound to heparin-like molecules on the cell surface or in the extracellular matrix.

Several of the cultured cell types investigated (e.g., fibroblasts and BCE cells) both produced bFGF and had high-affinity receptors for the molecule. This suggests that for some cells bFGF may act as an autocrine hormone.

ACKNOWLEDGMENTS

This work was supported by grants CA-34282 from the National Institutes of Health, CD-77 from the American Cancer Society, and 1811 from the Council for Tobacco Research, Inc. D.M. was supported by an investigatorship from the New York Heart Association.

REFERENCES
Gross, J.L., D. Moscatelli, and D.B. Rifkin. 1983. Increased capillary endothelial cell protease activity in response to angiogenic stimuli *in vitro*. *Proc. Natl. Acad. Sci.* **80**: 2623.
Moscatelli, D., M. Presta, and D.B. Rifkin. 1986a. Purification of a factor from human placenta that stimulates capillary endothelial cell protease production, DNA synthesis, and migration. *Proc. Natl. Acad. Sci.* **83**: 2091.

Moscatelli, D., M. Presta, J. Joseph-Silverstein, and D.B. Rifkin. 1986b. Both normal and tumor cells produce basic fibroblast growth factor. *J. Cell. Physiol.* **129**: 273.

Neufeld, G. and D. Gospodarowicz. 1985. The identification and partial characterization of the fibroblast growth factor receptor of baby hamster kidney cells. *J. Biol. Chem.* **260**: 13860.

Presta, M., D. Moscatelli, J. Joseph-Silverstein, and D.B. Rifkin. 1986. Purification from a human hepatoma cell line of a basic fibroblast growth factor-like molecule that stimulates capillary endothelial cell plasminogen activator production, DNA synthesis, and migration. *Mol. Cell. Biol.* **6**: 4060.

Eye-derived Growth Factors: Receptors and Early Event Studies

M. Moenner, J. Badet, B. Chevallier, M. Tardieu, J. Courty, and D. Barritault

Laboratoire de Biotechnologie des Cellules Eucaryotes
Universite de Paris Val de Marne, 94010 Creteil Cedex, France

Eye-derived growth factors I and II (EDGF I and II) have been purified from bovine retina (Barritault et al. 1982; Courty et al. 1985) and represent the two families of heparin-binding growth factors that have been purified to homogeneity by several groups in the last 2 years. We have shown that EDGF I corresponds to basic fibroblast growth factor (bFGF) (Courty et al. 1986) and that EDGF II corresponds to endothelial cell growth factor or acidic FGF (aFGF) (Schreiber et al. 1985).

Although the mitogenic properties of partially purified preparations have been described for over a decade (Armelin 1973; Gospodarowicz 1975), very little information on the mechanism of action of these growth factors is known. We have obtained highly purified preparations of aFGF and bFGF and have studied the interaction of these growth factors with target cells.

Characterization of High-affinity Receptors to EDGF I/bFGF

Binding and receptor studies were made possible by labeling conditions that maintained the growth factors biologically active. We were able to show (Moenner et al. 1986) that ^{125}I-labeled bFGF bound to bovine epithelial lens cells in culture could be displaced by unlabeled bFGF in a dose-dependent manner and that almost 90% of the radioactivity was displaced by a 100 molar excess of unlabeled bFGF. Scatchard analysis indicated an apparent dissociation constant of 5×10^{-11} M. Using cross-linking agents, we bound this growth factor to its putative receptor and could estimate an apparent M_r of 130,000 for this receptor.

Evidence for High- and Low-affinity Receptors

To purify the M_r 130,000 receptors, we looked for cells rich in receptors. The results are presented in Table 1. We also found that the number of high-affinity receptors could vary for the same cells, accord-

Table 1 High-affinity Specific Binding of aFGF (EDGF II) and bFGF (EDGF I) on Mammalian Cells

Cells	Cells/cm² ($\times 10^{-5}$)	aFGF sites/cell	Apparent K_d ($\text{M} \times 10^{10}$)	bFGF sites/cell	Apparent K_d ($\text{M} \times 10^{10}$)
Bovine epithelial lens	0.4			20,000	0.5
Baby hamster kidney (BHK-21)	2.8	30,000	7.0	15,000	6.0
Chinese hamster lung fibroblasts (CCL39)	0.9	10,000	1.0	50,000	1.0
	2.9			10,000	0.8
Mouse fibroblasts (BALB/3T3)	2.5			5,000	0.6
Human fibroblasts (AG1523)	0.2			100,000	0.5
Bovine endothelial cornea	0.4	12,000	0.5	10,000	0.9
Murine lung endothelial capillary (LE II)	0.4			15,000	0.3
Human epidermoid carcinoma A431	1.2	<1,000		<1,000	
Human alveolar carcinoma A549	2.5	<1,000		<1,000	

Binding was performed at 4°C. Nonspecific binding was determined in the presence of a large excess of partially purified FGF/EDGF (acidic acid extract; Barritault et al. 1982).

ing to cellular density. Scatchard analysis also indicated the existence of a second class of receptors (400,000 to 1,000,000 per cell) with an apparent dissociation constant of 1×10^{-9} to 2×10^{-9} M (not shown). Furthermore, preliminary experiments (not shown) indicated that this second class of receptors was partially sensitive to heparinase treatment but not to chondroitinase.

EDGF/FGF Does Not Induce Hydrolysis of Polyphosphoinositide

We have shown (Magnaldo et al. 1986) that the addition of aFGF or bFGF to bovine epithelial lens cells or Chinese hamster fibroblasts cells (CCL39) induces a rise of intracellular pH (0.2 to 0.4 units) and free-calcium concentration (240 nM to 400 nM). The origin of the

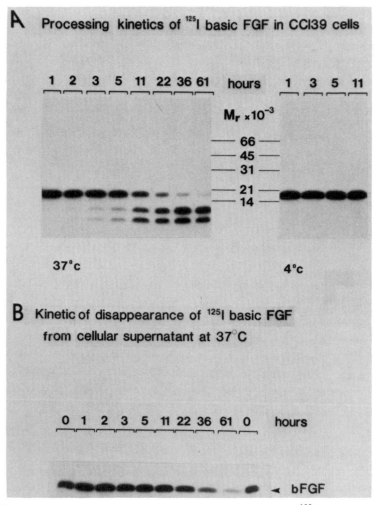

Figure 1 Autoradiograph of the electrophoretic migration of ^{125}I-labeled FGF associated with cellular extracts (A) and present in cellular supernatant (B) at different times of incubation at 37°C and 4°C. ^{125}I-labeled FGF was added at 5 ng/ml of culture medium.

calcium was strictly extracellular. Furthermore, the breakdown of phosphoinositide was not activated, suggesting that another pathway might be involved in the mitogenic response. This hypothesis is supported by a recent report that a tyrosine kinase activity might be associated with the FGF receptor (Huang and Huang 1986).

Processing of EDGF I/bFGF

Study of the fate of EDGF I/bFGF was carried out by the addition of ^{125}I-labeled bFGF to subconfluent G_0-arrested CCL39 cells maintained in serum-free medium. The doses of ^{125}I-labeled bFGF used ensured maximal stimulation of thymidine incorporation for these cells.

At different incubation times at 4°C and 37°C, the migration of ^{125}I-labeled bFGF associated with the cell lysate, as well as in the culture medium, was studied by gel electrophoresis. Autoradiographs of the electrophoretic migrations are shown in Figure 1. At 4°C, there is no detectable degradation in the cell medium. At 37°C, two faint degradation bands at 10 kD and 8 kD, associated with the cell lysate, are detectable after 2 hours of incubation. These bands become more visible as the incubation time increases. Concomitantly, the 17 kD (intact bFGF) band decreased in intensity in both the cell lysate and culture medium. The radioactivity associated with these bands was measured, and the results are presented in Table 2.

Table 2 Fate of ^{125}I-labeled bFGF Incubated with CCL39 Fibroblasts at 37°C

(a) Repartition of radioactivity in cellular supernatant (%)

Culture medium	Incubation time (hr)							
	1	2	3	5	11	22	36	61
Intact FGF (17K)	100	102	105	90	60	44	30	21
Degraded FGF	0	0	0	10	40	56	70	79

(b) Repartition of radioactivity associated with cells (%)

Cell extract	Incubation time (hr)							
	1	2	3	5	11	22	36	61
Intact FGF (17K)	100	82	72	65	40	25	13	5
10K fragment	0	3	14	15	32	42	54	54
8K fragment	0	3	14	15	27	29	30	32

Radioactivity was counted in the 17K, 10K, and 8K bands after electrophoresis (Fig. 1). Results are given as a percentage of the radioactivity loaded on each track of the gel.

55

DISCUSSION

Our results indicate that EDGFs/FGFs have most of the properties of other growth factors with regard to high-affinity receptors and mitogenic pathway. However, the processing is slow and depends on the formation of intermediate products. Further investigations are now in progress to characterize these intermediate products and to determine if they play a significant role in the mechanism of action of EDGF/bFGF.

In addition to study of its angiogenic activity, the wound-healing properties of EDGF have been studied in models of corneal and epidermal ulceration (Thompson et al. 1982; Fourtanier et al. 1986). It is therefore important to increase our understanding of the mechanism of action of these molecules in the control of cell division and tissue homeostasis in order to elucidate their physiological meaning as well as to use them as wound-healing agents.

ACKNOWLEDGMENTS

This work was supported by the Association pour la Recherche sur le Cancer, the Ligue Nationale contre le cancer, the Ministère de l'Education Nationale, the Ministère de la Recherche et Technologie, the A.T.P. 955 341 from the NCRS, and the association Naturalia et Biologia.

REFERENCES

Armelin, H.A. 1973. Pituitary extracts and steroid hormones in the control of 3T3 cell growth. *Proc. Natl. Acad. Sci.* **70**: 2702.

Barritault, D., J. Ploüet, J. Courty, and Y. Courtois. 1982. Purification, characterization and biological properties of the eye-derived growth factor from retina: Analogies with brain-derived growth factor. *J. Neurosci. Res.* **8**: 477.

Courty, J., C. Loret, M. Moenner, B. Chevallier, O. Lagente, Y. Courtois, and D. Barritault. 1985. Bovine retina contains three growth factor activities with different affinity to heparin: Eye-derived growth factor I, II, III. *Biochimie* **67**: 265.

Courty, J., B. Chevallier, M. Moenner, C. Loret, O. Lagente, P. Böhlen, Y. Courtois, and D. Barritault. 1986. Evidence for FGF-like growth factor in adult bovine retina: Analogies with EDGF I. *Biochem. Biophys. Res. Commun.* **136**: 102.

Fourtanier, A., J. Courty, E. Muller, Y. Courtois, M. Prunieras, and D. Barritault. 1986. Eye-derived growth factor isolated from bovine retina and used for epidermal wound healing *in vivo*. *J. Invest. Dermatol.* **87**: 76.

Gospodarowicz, D. 1975. Purification of a fibroblast growth factor from bovine pituitary. *J. Biol. Chem.* **87**: 2515.

Huang, S.S. and J.S. Huang. 1986. Association of bovine brain-derived growth factor receptor with protein tyrosine kinase activity. *J. Biol. Chem.* **261**: 9568.

Magnaldo, I., G. L'Allemain, J.C. Chambard, M. Moenner, D. Barritault, and J. Pouysségur. 1986. The mitogenic signaling pathway of fibroblast growth factor is not mediated through polyphosphoinositide hydrolysis and protein kinase C activation in hamster fibroblasts. *J. Biol. Chem.* **261**: 16916.

Moenner, M., B. Chevallier, J. Badet, and D. Barritault. 1986. Evidence and characterization of the receptor to eye-derived growth factor I, the retinal form of basic fibroblast growth factor, on bovine epithelial lens cells. *Proc. Natl. Acad. Sci.* **83**: 5024.

Schreiber, A.B., J. Kenney, J. Kowalski, K.A. Thomas, G. Gimenez-Gallego, M. Rios-Candelore, M. Di Salvo, D. Barritault, J. Courty, Y. Courtois, M. Moenner, O. Loret, W.H. Burgess, T. Mehlmann, R. Friesel, W. Johnson, and T. Maciag. 1985. A unique family of endothelial cell polypeptide mitogens: The antigenic and receptor cross-reactivity of bovine endothelial cell growth factor, brain-derived acidic fibroblast growth factor and eye-derived growth factor II. *J. Cell Biol.* **101**: 1623.

Thompson, P., J.M. Desbordes, J. Giraud, D. Barritault, Y. Pouliquen, and Y. Courtois. 1982. The effect of an eye-derived growth factor (EDGF) on corneal epithelial regeneration. *Exp. Eye Res.* **34**: 191.

Heparin-binding Endothelial Cell Growth Factors Are Sequestered by the Extracellular Matrix

I. Vlodavsky,* J. Folkman,[†‡] and M. Klagsbrun[†**]

*Department of Oncology, Hadassah-Hebrew University Hospital
Jerusalem 91120, Israel

[†]Department of Surgery, Children's Hospital
Boston, Massachusetts 02115

Departments of [‡]Anatomy and **Biological Chemistry
Harvard Medical School, Boston, Massachusetts 02115

Cultured bovine endothelial cells lay down an extracellular matrix (ECM) that replaces the requirement that various cell types have for fibroblast growth factor (FGF) in order for them to proliferate and express their differentiated functions (Gospodarowicz et al. 1980). The possible involvement of ECM-bound growth factors in the induction of cell proliferation has been minimized because ECM treated so as to inactivate growth factors still supports cell growth (Gospodarowicz et al. 1983). However, the possibility that ECM contains highly stable growth factors has not been fully ruled out.

Recently, it has been shown that angiogenic FGF-like growth factors have a strong affinity for heparin (Shing et al. 1984) and are also synergized (Thornton et al. 1983), protected, and stabilized (Gospodarowicz and Cheng 1986) by heparin. The presence of heparan sulfate as the major glycosaminoglycan in the subendothelial ECM (Robinson and Gospodarowicz 1983) raised the possibility that ECM contains heparin-binding endothelial cell growth factors that are tightly bound and possibly stabilized by the ECM heparan sulfate. In this paper, we show that endothelial cells synthesize heparin-binding basic FGF (bFGF), most of which remains cell-associated and some of which is deposited and sequestered in the subendothelial ECM. Heparin-binding growth factors that are structurally and functionally related to bFGF are also stored in the ECM of the bovine cornea in vivo, mainly in Descemet's membrane.

RESULTS
Endothelial-cell-derived bFGF-like Growth Factors
Extracts of cultured bovine aortic and corneal endothelial cells were

58

analyzed by heparin-Sepharose affinity chromatography for growth factor activity. A single growth factor peak eluted from the column at about 1.5 M NaCl and comigrated with hepatoma-derived (Klagsbrun et al. 1986) and brain-derived bFGFs. The active fractions were highly mitogenic for bovine aortic and capillary endothelial cells. Antibodies to synthetic peptides corresponding to both the amino-terminal and internal regions of pituitary bFGF cross-reacted in electrophoretic transfer (Western) blots with a polypeptide doublet (m.w. 18,400) purified from endothelial cell lysates by heparin-Sepharose chromatography. Biosynthesis of bFGF was demonstrated by metabolic labeling of endothelial cell cultures followed by immunoprecipitation with anti-bFGF sera, SDS-PAGE, and fluorography, as described previously (Klagsbrun et al. 1986). The anti-bFGF sera, but not preimmune sera, immunoprecipitated an 18,400-dalton polypeptide (Vlodavsky et al. 1987b).

Extraction of bFGF-like Growth Factors from the Subendothelial ECM

Extracts of ECM prepared with 2 M NaCl or collagenase digestion stimulated the growth of aortic (Fig. 1a) and capillary endothelial cells, regardless of whether the ECM was exposed by lysing the cells with Triton/NH$_4$OH (Gospodarowicz et al. 1980) or by treatment with 1 M urea involving little or no cell lysis (Gospodarowicz et al. 1983). These results indicate that most of the matrix-associated growth-promoting activity represented growth factor deposited by viable cells into ECM rather than by lysed cells. Heparin-Sepharose chromatography of ECM extracts yielded a single peak of growth factor eluting at about 1.5 M NaCl (Fig. 1a). When a sample of this peak was analyzed by electrophoretic transfer blot, anti-bFGF sera cross-reacted with a polypeptide doublet with a molecular weight of about 18,400 (Fig. 1b, lane 1), suggesting that the matrix-derived growth factor was a form of bFGF.

Descemet's Membrane Contains a Potent Heparin-binding Growth Factor for Capillary Endothelial Cells

Although the cornea is normally avascular, injury to Descemet's membrane can induce intense neovascularization. This suggested to us that Descemet's membrane, like the subendothelial ECM deposited in vitro, contains sequestered angiogenic factors. Bovine corneas were dissected into three layers. The inner layer, comprising almost pure Descemet's membrane, was found to contain large quantities of readily releasable, angiogenic, heparin-binding growth factors for capillary endothelial cells. These factors appeared to be structurally related to bFGF by the criteria that they (1) eluted from heparin-Sepharose at 1.6–1.7 M NaCl,

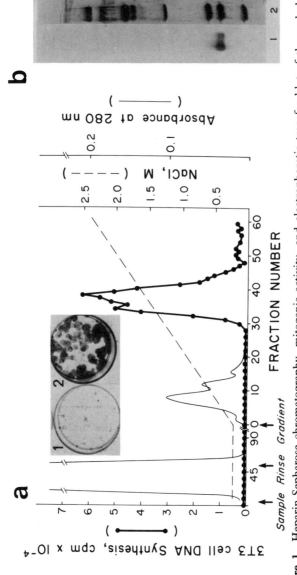

Figure 1 Heparin-Sepharose chromatography, mitogenic activity, and electrophoretic transfer blot of the endothelial cell matrix-derived growth factor. (*a*) Heparin-Sepharose chromatography. ECM coated 10-cm culture dishes were digested with collagenase; the extract was applied to a column of heparin-Sepharose, and growth factor activity was eluted with a gradient of 0.1–2.5 M NaCl. (*Insert*) Mitogenic activity. Bovine aortic endothelial cells were seeded at a clonal density in the absence (*1*) or presence (*2*) of a dialyzed 2 M NaCl extract of ECM; 14 days after seeding, cultures were fixed and cell colonies were strained with 0.1% Crystal Violet. (*b*) Electrophoretic transfer blot. Active fractions eluted from heparin-Sepharose were dialyzed, lyophilized, and electrophoresed on SDS-PAGE. Proteins were transferred to nitrocellulose and stained with an antibody directed against a synthetic peptide representing an internal sequence of bFGF (lane *1*).

(2) had a molecular weight of about 18,000, (3) cross-reacted with antibodies against bFGF when analyzed by electrophoretic blotting and immunofluorescence, and (4) were potent mitogens for bovine capillary endothelial cells. When the three corneal layers were subjected to more extensive extraction conditions, heparin-binding bFGF-like growth factors were released also from the middle (stromal) and outer (epithelial) portions of the cornea, albeit at smaller amounts as compared with that of Descemet's membrane. Immunofluorescence studies using affinity-purified anti-bFGF antibodies confirmed that FGF-like growth factors were concentrated mainly in Descemet's membrane in vivo.

These findings indicate that Descemet's membrane and, to a lesser extent, other parts of the cornea may serve as a physiological depot for storage of angiogenic molecules. Abnormal release of these factors could be responsible for a variety of different types of pathological corneal neovascularization (J. Folkman et al., in prep.).

Medium Conditioned by Bovine Aortic Endothelial Cells Contains PDGF-like but not FGF-like Growth Factors

Bovine aortic endothelial cells were cultured in a medium containing serum depleted of platelet-derived growth factor (PDGF), prepared by two cycles of chromatography over heparin-Sepharose. Whereas control medium containing serum depleted of PDGF yielded no detectable growth factor activity, the endothelial cell conditioned medium had a high mitogenic activity eluting from heparin-Sepharose at about 0.4 M NaCl, but little or no growth factor activity eluting at a high (1.4–1.6 M) concentration of salt. Growth factor eluting at 0.4 M NaCl was, like PDGF, sensitive to dithiothreitol and resistant to heat, guanidine HCl, and low pH. In addition, it competed with PDGF for binding to fibroblasts and had no mitogenic activity on capillary endothelial cells (Vlodavsky et al. 1987a).

Sequestration of Hepatoma-derived bFGF by the ECM Heparan Sulfate

Since heparan sulfate constitutes more than 90% of the subendothelial ECM glycosaminoglycan side chains (Robinson and Gospodarowicz 1983), it is likely that heparin-binding growth factors such as bFGF are sequestered by means of high-affinity binding to heparan sulfate. Evidence for such binding was obtained in studies on the interaction of hepatoma-derived bFGF (Klagsbrun et al. 1986) with the subendothelial ECM. It was found that hepatoma-derived bFGF binds to ECM and can be released by incubation with either 2 M NaCl, heparan sulfate, heparin, or various heparin fragments as small as the disaccharide. Degradation of the ECM heparan sulfate by heparanase, and to a lesser extent by heparinase, as well as digestion of the matrix with trypsin or collagenase, released the ECM-bound hepatoma-derived bFGF. In contrast, there was little or no release of growth-promoting activity upon incubation of the ECM with hyaluronic acid, chondroitin sulfate, or chondroitinase ABC (Table 1). Thus, heparan sulfate in the ECM may serve as a sink to concentrate and stabilize heparin-binding growth factors in the vicinity of cell-surface receptors and may provide an indirect pathway for induction of angiogenesis by cells capable of releasing the matrix-sequestered angiogenic factors.

DISCUSSION

The present study demonstrated that endothelial cells synthesize a bFGF-like growth factor, most of which remains cell-associated but up to 30% of which is deposited and sequestered by the subendothelial ECM. Endothelial cells also synthesize a PDGF-like growth factor that, unlike FGF, is secreted into the growth medium and is not readily detected in either cell lysate or subendothelial ECM. Whereas the readily secreted PDGF-like factor may exert a paracrine function on neighboring cells of the vessel wall, the cell-associated bFGF-like factor may fulfill an autocrine function restricted to the repair of the vascular endothelium in response to an endothelial cell perturbation or injury.

Table 1 Release of ECM-sequestered Hepatoma-derived bFGF

Treatment	3T3 cell DNA synthesis ([^{3}H]thymidine, cpm)
Glycosaminoglycans	
control	3,188
heparin	38,284
heparan sulfate	46,424
chondroitin sulfate	4,692
hyaluronic acid	3,640
Enzymes	
chondroitinase ABC (0.5 μ/ml)	4,798
heparinase (0.1 μ/ml)	33,794
heparanase (0.1 μ/ml)	108,898
trypsin (20 μg/ml)	123,886
collagenase (20 μg/ml)	145,854

ECM-coated wells (16 mm) were incubated (6 hr, 4°C) with hepatoma-derived bFGF (10 units/well) in PBS containing 0.15% BSA. The ECM was washed 5 times with RPMI medium to remove the unbound factor and incubated (3 hr, 4°C) with the various glycosaminoglycans (10 μg/ml) or enzymes. Aliquots (10–40 μl) of the incubation mixture were tested for stimulation of [^{3}H]thymidine incorporation into the DNA of quiesent 3T3 cells.

The lack of bFGF release into culture medium is consistent with recent studies on the gene structure of both basic and acidic FGFs, indicating that they both lack a signal peptide (Abraham et al. 1986; Jaye et al. 1986). One possibility for the activity of these factors on other cells may be leakage due to cell damage and dysfunction. An alternative pathway may be that a substantial amount of FGF is directed through the basal cell surface into the subcellular ECM, perhaps in association with heparan sulfate. It remains to be investigated whether FGF-like factors form an intracellular and/or extracellular complex with heparan sulfate and whether they remain associated with fragments of heparan sulfate after being released from ECM. In support of the latter possibility is the release of ECM-bound FGF-like factors by treatment with heparanase. If the results of these studies apply to ECM in vivo, then heparanase activity in certain tumor cells and inflammatory cells (Vlodavsky et al. 1985) is likely to be indirectly involved in the induction of angiogenesis. ECM storage of growth factors and other biologically active molecules may stabilize and potentiate their activity so as to allow a more persistent effect at a given location and time, as compared with the same molecules in a fluid phase.

ACKNOWLEDGMENTS
This work was supported by National Cancer Institute grants CA-30289 (to I.V.), CA-37392 (to M.K.), and CA-14019 (to J.F.).

REFERENCES
Abraham, J.A., A. Mergia, J.L. Whang, A. Tumolo, J. Friedman, K.A. Hjerrild, D. Gospodarowicz, and J.C. Fiddes. 1986. Nucleotide sequence of a bovine clone encoding the angiogenic protein, basic fibroblast growth factor. *Science* **233**: 545.

Gospodarowicz, D. and J. Cheng. 1986. Heparin protects basic and acidic FGF from inactivation. *J. Cell. Physiol.* **128**: 475.

Gospodarowicz, D., R. Gonzalez, and D.K. Fujii. 1983. Are factors originating from serum, plasma, or cultured cells involved in the growth-promoting effect of the extracellular matrix produced by cultured bovine corneal endothelial cells? *J. Cell. Physiol.* **114**: 191.

Gospodarowicz, D., I. Vlodavsky, and N. Savion. 1980. The extracellular matrix and the control of proliferation of vascular endothelial and vascular smooth muscle cells. *J. Supramol. Struct.* **13**: 339.

Jaye, M., R. Howk, W. Burgess, G.A. Ricca, I.M. Chiu, M.W. Ravera, S.J. O'Brien, W.S. Modi, T. Maciag, and W.N. Droham. 1986. Human endothelial cell growth factor: Cloning, nucleotide sequence and chromosome localization. *Science* **233**: 541.

Klagsbrun, M., J. Sasse, R. Sullivan, and J.A. Smith. 1986. Human tumor cells synthesize an endothelial cell growth factor that is structurally related to basic fibroblast growth factor. *Proc. Natl. Acad. Sci.* **83**: 2448.

Robinson, J. and D. Gospodarowicz. 1983. Glycoaminoglycans synthesized by bovine corneal endothelial cells in culture. *J. Cell. Physiol.* **117**: 368.

Shing, Y., J. Folkman, R. Sullivan, C. Butterfield, J. Murray, and M. Klagsbrun. 1984. Heparin affinity: Purification of a tumor-derived capillary endothelial cell growth factor. *Science* **223**: 1296.

Thornton, S.C., S.N. Mueller, and E.M. Levine. 1983. Human endothelial cells: Use of heparin in cloning and long term serial cultivation. *Science* **222**: 623.

Vlodavsky, I., R. Fridman, R. Sullivan, J. Sasse, and M. Klagsbrun. 1987a. Aortic endothelial cells synthesize basic fibroblast growth factor which remains cell-associated and platelet-derived growth factor-like protein which is secreted. *J. Cell Physiol.* (in press).

Vlodavsky, I., J. Folkman, R. Sullivan, R. Fridman, R. Ishai-Michaeli, J. Sasse, and M. Klagsbrun. 1987b. Endothelial cell-derived basic fibroblast growth factor; synthesis and deposition into subendothelial extracellular matrix. *Proc. Natl. Acad. Sci.* (in press).

Vlodavsky, I., Z. Fuks, M. Bar-Ner, J. Yahalom, A. Eldor, N. Savion, J. Naparstek, I.R. Cohen, M. Kramer, and V. Schirrmacher. 1985. Degradation of heparan sulfate in the subendothelial basement membrane by normal and malignant blood borne cells. In *Extracellular matrix: Structure and function* (ed. K.A. Piez and A.H. Reddi), p. 283. Elsevier, New York.

Production of Platelet-derived Growth Factor-like Protein by Endothelial Cells

P.E. DiCorleto, P.L. Fox, and G.M. Chisolm
Department of Brain and Vascular Research
Cleveland Clinic Research Institute
Cleveland, Ohio 44106

The endothelium is no longer thought to function solely as a passive barrier between the blood and tissue. The fact that many biologically active molecules are produced in endothelial cells (ECs) suggests that this cell plays an active role in such physiological processes as vessel development and remodeling, wound healing, formation of collateral circulation, vessel contraction and relaxation, and immune system responses. Bovine aortic ECs were the first proliferative diploid cell found to secrete mitogenic activity for fibroblasts (3T3 cells) and smooth-muscle cells (Gajdusek et al. 1980). Since that time, cultured vascular ECs from many species and sources have been shown to secrete growth factors for connective-tissue cells constitutively. Levels of mitogen are sufficiently high that smooth-muscle cells or fibroblasts, when cocultured with ECs in the absence of exogenous mitogens, will proliferate as if in the presence of a high concentration of serum. The growth-promoting activity in EC-conditioned media can be separated into two major mitogens, one of which, designated PDGFc[1] and comprising approximately 25% of the total, is biochemically and immunologically indistinguishable from platelet-derived growth factor (PDGF) (DiCorleto and Bowen-Pope 1983). A second major mitogen in the EC-conditioned media does not bind to the PDGF receptor on fibroblasts, is not recognized by antibody to PDGF, and is biochemically separable from PDGF (DiCorleto 1984).

The observation that the B-chain of PDGF is homologous to the product of the c-*sis* gene led to the cloning of the EC c-*sis* gene from a human EC cDNA library (Collins et al. 1985). Several investigators have quantitated c-*sis* (PDGF) mRNA in cultured ECs, and one group (Barrett et al. 1984) compared levels in vitro to those present in freshly isolated bovine aortic and human umbilical vein ECs. The "in vivo"

---

[1] "c" refers to the ability of this protein to compete for binding to the PDGF receptor.

65

ECs demonstrated 10-fold to 100-fold less c-*sis* mRNA than did their cultured counterparts. These data suggest that PDGF production is regulatable and raise the possibility that certain pathological conditions may mimic culture conditions and lead to an inappropriate production of mitogens.

Stimulators of PDGFc Production by Endothelium
The production of PDGFc by cultured ECs can be stimulated by several exogenous factors. We have reported that certain chemicals that are injurious to bovine aortic ECs, including lethal doses of bacterial endotoxin and phorbol esters, stimulate production of PDGFc (Fox and DiCorleto 1984). A slowly dying cell was found to release as much of this mitogen as did a healthy cell in 19 days, whereas ECs that were rapidly killed by freeze-thaw cycles or hypotonic lysis released negligible levels of PDGFc. The latter result indicates that ECs possess a small intracellular pool of this mitogen in a receptor-bindable state and that the increased production in the presence of the injurious agents is not due solely to cell lysis. Proliferation of cultured ECs did not affect production of PDGFc; the rate of secretion per cell was the same for rapidly dividing and confluent, quiescent cells. "Quiescent" ECs in culture, however, have a far higher turnover rate than ECs in vivo, and therefore it is possible that truly quiescent cultured ECs may exhibit reduced production of PDGFc, similar to freshly isolated ECs.

Harlan et al. (1986) have reported that incubation of human umbilical vein ECs with physiological concentrations of human α-thrombin, a protease that may be present at sites of inflammation, resulted in fivefold stimulation of production of PDGFc in 24 hours. Unlike in our experiments with endotoxin and phorbol esters, α-thrombin did not affect cell viability; furthermore, the stimulated production of PDGFc was not prevented by cycloheximide, indicating that posttranslational modification of an inactive precursor may be involved. Gajdusek et al. (1986) have reported a similar finding in EC cultures treated with factor Xa. These studies indicate that vessel injury and its repair process may result in the aberrant production of paracrine growth factors by the endothelium.

Inhibitors of PDGFc Production by Endothelium
Endothelial production of PDGFc by cultured cells can also be suppressed by specific culture conditions. Jaye et al. (1985) showed that the organization of human umbilical vein ECs into tubular structures was accompanied by decreased expression of mRNA for the B-chain of PDGF. Substratum composition may also influence growth factor production by ECs. Bovine aortic ECs plated on Vitrogen (bovine dermal

collagen type I; Flow Laboratories) initially produced low levels of PDGFc, compared to cells plated on plastic or fibronectin-treated plastic (DiCorleto and Chisolm 1986). The production rate returned to control levels after 5 days. We have recently reported that low-density lipoprotein (LDL) modified by acetylation (acetyl-LDL) or reaction with dimethylpropanediamine, but not native LDL, inhibited production of PDGFc by bovine aortic ECs (Fox and DiCorleto 1986). The decreased production (to 1–25% of control level) was specific, since total cellular and secreted protein syntheses were unaffected by either modified lipoprotein. Human umbilical vein ECs were similarly regulated by acetyl-LDL, but a line of rat heart ECs was not. These results are consistent with the presence of active scavenger (acetyl-LDL) receptors, since bovine aortic and human umbilical vein ECs have this receptor, whereas rat heart ECs do not.

We have recently determined that the inhibitory molecule in the acetyl-LDL is not cholesterol, since incubation of bovine aortic ECs with cholesterol/albumin complexes resulted in cellular loading of cholesterol but did not affect the production of PDGFc (Fox et al. 1986). By quantitating cholesterol esterification in the ECs, we verified that the cholesterol from the complexes, similar to that from acetyl-LDL, was entering a metabolically active intracellular pool. The regulatory molecular species has not yet been identified, but we have evidence that it is peroxidized lipid, since (1) native LDL oxidized in vitro also specifically inhibited production of PDGFc, (2) the ability of acetyl-LDL to inhibit production was dependent on its oxidation level, and (3) lipid extracted from oxidized LDL, but not native LDL, inhibited production.

We have begun studies to elucidate the mechanism of action of the inhibitory lipid. Chloroquine, monensin, and NH_4Cl, inhibitors of lysosomal hydrolytic activity, did not prevent acetyl-LDL-mediated inhibition of PDGFc production, indicating that cellular metabolism of the lipoprotein was not required for the inhibition. Furthermore, acetyl-LDL suppressed PDGFc production by ECs even in the presence of butylated hydroxytoluene, an inhibitor of lipid peroxidation, suggesting that cellular propagation of free radicals was not required for the inhibition. Finally, inhibition of PDGFc production is likely to be posttranscriptional, since Northern blot analysis using a v-*sis* probe showed that the PDGF B-chain mRNA levels were unaffected by oxidized or acetylated LDL.

SIGNIFICANCE

Cultured ECs can be activated to release PDGFc by injurious agents and by components of the coagulation cascade. Our recent findings indicate that PDGFc production by ECs is specifically and markedly suppressed by a component of oxidized lipoproteins. These results suggest the possibility that humoral and arterial factors may affect the functional state of ECs in vivo and thus influence the role of the endothelium in normal and pathological processes. An understanding of the regulation of EC growth factor production may suggest ways to restore dysfunctional cells to the normal state.

ACKNOWLEDGMENTS

These studies were supported by National Institutes of Health grant HL-29582 (to G.M.C. and P.E.D.) and by a Grant-in-Aid from the American Heart Association, Northeast Ohio Affiliate (to P.L.F.). P.E.D. is the recipient of a Research Career Development Award (HL-01561) from the National Institutes of Health.

REFERENCES

Barrett, T.B., C.M. Gajdusek, S.M. Schwartz, J.K. McDougall, and E.P. Benditt. 1984. Expression of the *sis* gene by endothelial cells in culture and *in vivo*. *Proc. Natl. Acad. Sci.* **81:** 6772.

Collins, T., D. Ginsburg, J.M. Boss, S.H. Orkin, and J.S. Pober. 1985. Cultured human endothelial cells express platelet-derived growth factor B chain: cDNA cloning and structural analysis. *Nature* **316:** 748.

DiCorleto, P.E. 1984. Cultured endothelial cells produce multiple growth factors for connective tissue cells. *Exp. Cell Res.* **153:** 167.

DiCorleto, P.E. and D.F. Bowen-Pope. 1983. Cultured endothelial cells produce a platelet-derived growth factor-like protein. *Proc. Natl. Acad. Sci.* **80:** 1919.

DiCorleto, P.E., and G.M. Chisolm III. 1986. Participation of the endothelium in the development of the atherosclerotic plaque. *Prog. Lipid Res.* (in press).

Fox, P.L. and P.E. DiCorleto. 1984. Regulation of production of a platelet-derived growth factor-like protein by cultured bovine aortic endothelial cells. *J. Cell. Physiol.* **121:** 298.

———. 1986. Modified low density lipoproteins suppress production of a platelet-derived growth factor-like protein by cultured endothelial cells. *Proc. Natl. Acad. Sci.* **83:** 4774.

Fox, P.L., G.M. Chisolm, and P.E. DiCorleto. 1986. Inhibition of endothelial production of PDGF-like protein by acetylated LDL depends on lipid peroxidation. *Arteriosclerosis* **6:** 562a (Abstr.).

Gajdusek, C., P. DiCorleto, R. Ross, and S.M. Schwartz. 1980. An endothelial cell-derived growth factor. *J. Cell Biol.* **85:** 467.

Gajdusek, C.M., S. Carbon, R. Ross, P. Nawroth, and D. Stern. 1986. Activation of coagulation releases endothelial cell mitogens. *J. Cell Biol.* **101:** 419.

Harlan, J.M., P.J. Thompson, R. Ross, and D.F. Bowen-Pope. 1986. α-Thrombin induces release of platelet-derived growth factor-like molecule(s) by cultured human endothelial cells. *J. Cell Biol.* **103:** 1129.

Jaye, M., E. McConathy, W. Drohan, B. Tong, T. Deuel, and T. Maciag. 1985. Modulation of the *sis* gene transcript during endothelial cell differentiation in vitro. *Science* **228:** 882.

Transforming Growth Factor-β: Stimulator or Inhibitor of Angiogenesis?

A.B. Roberts and M.B. Sporn

Laboratory of Chemoprevention, National Cancer Institute
Bethesda, Maryland 20892

Transforming growth factor-β (TGF-β) has been shown to be a potent inducer of angiogenesis in vivo. In the rabbit cornea, 1–10 ng of TGF-β induces angiogenesis, and subcutaneous injection of 800 ng/day in newborn mice induces new blood vessel formation in 3 days. In each of these model systems, the angiogenic response is accompanied by inflammation, stromal thickening, and collagen synthesis. In contrast to its effects in vivo, TGF-β is consistently inhibitory to growth of endothelial cells in vitro, whether the cells are grown on plastic, on basement-membrane constituents, or on collagen gels. It also inhibits the stimulatory effects of fibroblast growth factor and phorbol myristate acetate on endothelial cells in vitro. This lack of a direct in vitro stimulation of endothelial cell growth and the demonstrated chemotactic activity of TGF-β for monocytes and its ability to stimulate monocytes to secrete factors mitogenic for fibroblasts suggest that the observed in vivo angiogenic activity of TGF-β might be mediated, in part, through its effects on recruitment of monocytes/macrophages and activation of these cells to secrete putative angiogenic factors.

TGF-β is a homodimeric peptide (m.w. 25,000) found principally in platelets and in bone. Although discovered and purified on the basis of its ability to induce anchorage-independent growth of certain fibroblastic cells ("transformation"), this peptide is now known to elicit many different biologic effects on a wide spectrum of target cells, including stimulation or inhibition of growth, stimulation or inhibition of differentiation, and modulation of cell function (for review, see Roberts and Sporn 1985; Sporn et al. 1986). The action of TGF-β is distinct from that of mitogenic peptides such as epidermal growth factor, platelet-derived growth factor, and interleukin-2; the effects of TGF-β on the growth of cells in vitro are often inhibitory and antagonistic to the effects of many other mitogens. Some of the actions of TGF-β may be mediated through its ability to stimulate the synthesis of matrix proteins including collagen and fibronectin (Ignotz and Massagué 1986; Roberts et al. 1986).

TGF-β Stimulates Angiogenesis In Vivo

Platelets, macrophages, and lymphocytes, three cell types involved in inflammation and repair processes, all have been shown to secrete TGF-β when activated (Sporn and Roberts 1986). Supporting these data, assay of wound fluid at various times following the insertion of wire-mesh Schilling-Hunt chambers into the backs of rats suggests that TGF-β might be an intrinsic mediator of the healing process; TGF-β levels increase about eightfold and reach maximum concentration (600 pM) in the wound fluid approximately 8–10 days after insertion of the chamber (D.T. Cromack et al., in prep.) In other experiments, exogenous addition of TGF-β by subcutaneous injection into the nape of the neck of newborn mice caused formation of granulation tissue (both an angiogenic and fibrotic response) similar to that seen in physiological wound healing (Roberts et al. 1986). These effects, which are reversible, occur 2–3 days after injection of 800 ng per animal.

TGF-β (1–10 ng) also induces the growth of new blood vessels when implanted into the rabbit cornea (V. Fiegel and D. Knighton, unpubl.). However, distinct from the effects of other angiogenic factors, TGF-β also caused an opacification of the cornea around the area of the implant. Histological examination revealed stromal thickening, collagen deposition, and large numbers of infiltrating mononuclear cells, similar to the effects of TGF-β injected subcutaneously into mice.

TGF-β Inhibits Angiogenesis In Vitro

In vitro, TGF-β inhibits the growth of endothelial cells whether those cells are grown on plastic, on basement-membrane components, or on collagen gels. TGF-β antagonizes the proliferation of both aortic (Fràter-Schröder et al. 1986) and capillary endothelial cells (Baird and Durkin 1986) induced by fibroblast growth factor (half-maximal inhibition at 4–20 pM). In capillary endothelial cells cultured on basement-membrane components, TGF-β also inhibits growth on laminin and type IV collagen (J. Madri, unpubl.). In capillary endothelial cells grown on type I collagen gels, TGF-β (200–400 pM) prevents the invasion and tubule formation that occurs after treatment with phorbol myristate acetate (R. Montesano, unpubl.).

Macrophages as Potential Mediators of the Angiogenic Effects of TGF-β

In vivo, TGF-β induces both angiogenesis and fibrosis. The effects on collagen and fibronectin synthesis are direct and are easily demonstrated in a variety of in vitro systems (Ignotz and Massagué 1986; Roberts et al. 1986). However, from the discussion above it is clear that the angiogenic effects of TGF-β in vivo are opposite to its effects on

70

endothelial cell growth in vitro. Given that there are limitations to these in vitro model systems, the data thus far suggest that effects of TGF-β on angiogenesis might be indirect and might be mediated by its effects on other cells.

TGF-β is an extremely potent chemotactic agent for human peripheral blood monocytes at concentrations ranging from 0.04 pM to 0.4 pM (S.M. Wahl et al., in prep.). At higher concentrations (>40 pM), TGF-β activates monocytes to secrete factors that are mitogenic for fibroblasts; whether some of these factors might also be mitogenic for endothelial cells has not yet been tested.

CONCLUSIONS

The inability to demonstrate a direct effect of TGF-β on the growth of endothelial cells in vitro in several different model systems suggests that its potent effects on angiogenesis in vivo might be mediated in part via effects on other cell types. The effects of TGF-β on monocyte chemotaxis and activation make these cells likely candidates to act as mediators of this response.

ACKNOWLEDGMENTS

We thank Drs. Roberto Montesano, Joseph Madri, Vance Fiegel, and David Knighton for sharing their unpublished data on the effects of TGF-β on angiogenic model systems.

REFERENCES

Baird, A. and T. Durkin. 1986. Inhibition of endothelial cell proliferation by type beta transforming growth factor: Interactions with acidic and basic fibroblast growth factors. *Biochem. Biophys. Res. Commun.* **138:** 476.

Fráter-Schröder, M., G. Müller, W. Birchmeier, and P. Böhlen. 1986. Transforming growth factor-beta inhibits endothelial cell proliferation. *Biochem. Biophys. Res. Commun.* **137:** 295.

Ignotz, R.A. and J. Massagué. 1986. Transforming growth factor beta stimulates the expression of fibronectin and collagen and their incorporation into the extra cellular matrix. *J. Biol. Chem.* **261:** 4337.

Roberts, A.B. and M.B. Sporn. 1985. Transforming growth factors. *Cancer Surv.* **4:** 683.

Roberts, A.B., M.B. Sporn, R.K. Assoian, J.M. Smith, N.S. Roche, L.M. Wakefield, U.I. Heine, L.A. Liotta, V. Falanga, J.H. Kehrl, and A.S. Fauci. 1986. Transforming growth factor beta: Rapid induction of fibrosis and angiogenesis in vivo and stimulation of collagen formation in vitro. *Proc. Natl. Acad. Sci.* **83:** 4167.

Sporn, M.B. and A.B. Roberts. 1986. Peptide growth factors and inflammation, tissue repair, and cancer. *J. Clin. Invest.* **78:** 329.

Sporn, M.B., A.B. Roberts, L.M. Wakefield, and R.K. Assoian. 1986. Transforming growth factor beta: Biological function and chemical structure. *Science* **233:** 532.

Transforming Growth Factor-α Induces Angiogenesis

R. Derynck,* M.E. Winkler,[†] and A.B. Schreiber[‡]**

Departments of *Molecular Biology and [†]Biocatalysis, Genentech, Inc.
South San Francisco, California 94080
[‡]Institute of Biological Sciences, Syntex Research
Palo Alto, California 94304

Transforming growth factors (TGFs) are polypeptides that can confer phenotypic transformation to several normal cells (DeLarco and Todaro 1978). TGF-α binds to the receptor for epidermal growth factor (EGF) and has been isolated from a variety of tumor cells (Todaro et al. 1985). TGF-β, which is not structurally related to TGF-α, binds to a distinct receptor and is synthesized by many normal and tumor cells (Anzano et al. 1982; Derynck et al. 1987). When fully processed, TGF-α and EGF display a 35% homology with conservation of all six cysteine residues (Derynck et al. 1984; Marquardt et al. 1984). The ability of EGF and TGF-α to bind to the same receptor (Massague 1983) is presumably due to the similarity in disulfide conformation (Marquardt et al. 1984). Although both peptides trigger many biological effects in a similar manner, they also differ in some of their activities, e.g., in the promotion of calcium release from fetal rat long bones in vitro, with TGF-α being more potent than EGF (Stern et al. 1985; Ibbotson et al. 1986). TGF-α is synthesized in embryos during early fetal development (Lee et al. 1985), in several virally transformed cells (Todaro et al. 1985), and in a large variety of human tumors (Derynck et al. 1987). It may play a role in neoplastic pathogenesis through an autocrine growth regulation mechanism (Sporn and Todaro 1980).

We have recently examined the expression of TGF-α in a large variety of human tumors and tumor cell lines (Derynck et al. 1987). Our data indicated that hematopoietic tumor cell lines lack TGF-α expression, whereas a large number of solid tumors express the TGF-α gene. The TGF-α expression appeared to be most prevalent in carcinomas. All renal and squamous carcinoma samples contained TGF-α mRNA, and TGF-α expression was also frequently seen in mammary

**Present addresses: Meloy Laboratories, Inc., Division of Immunology and Biologics, 6715 Electronic Drive, Springfield, Virginia 22151.

carcinomas and melanomas. The lack of TGF-α mRNA in hematopoietic tumors cells and the presence of it in many solid tumors, which depend on neovascularization for their development, prompted us to compare TGF-α and EGF for their ability to promote angiogenesis (Schreiber et al. 1986).

TGF-α Is More Angiogenic Than EGF

Human TGF-α was isolated from *Escherichia coli* containing a properly engineered plasmid (Derynck et al. 1984; Winkler et al. 1986) and was compared for its biological activities with natural mouse EGF. Both peptides were purified to apparent homogeneity as assessed by high-pressure liquid chromatography. The affinity of TGF-α was found to be 0.55 that of EGF for binding to the EGF receptor in CCL64 mink lung cells (Winkler et al. 1986). TGF-α and EGF, expressed as EGF-receptor-binding equivalents, were compared for their binding to the cell-surface receptors on four different cell types in culture: the A431 epidermoid carcinoma cell line, primary human foreskin fibroblasts, bovine pulmonary endothelial cells, and the murine lung microvascular endothelial cell line LEII. No significant differences were observed between the relative binding of both factors to these different cell types. Also, both growth factors were equally potent in inducing mitosis and induced a similar maximal mitogenic response in these cells (Schreiber et al. 1986). This effect was not measured in the A431 cells, which are known not to be mitogenically stimulated by these growth factors.

The growth factors were then compared for their angiogenic effects in vivo. For this experiment, we used a hamster cheek pouch bioassay, which allows the peptides to be prepared in physiological solvents for administration. The growth factors were mixed at different doses (0.3, 1, 3, and 10 μg) with blue agarose beads and infected subcutaneously in the pouch. These agarose beads serve as a nondenaturing form of a slow peptide-release system and mark the site of injection. Separate experiments with ^{125}I-labeled growth factors indicated that the rates of release of the two growth factors were very similar. The extent of angiogenesis in the hamster cheek pouch was assessed by subjective scoring on a scale from 0 (no new blood vessels) to 4 (many new tortuous vessels and hemorrhages in areas removed from the injection site) (Fig. 1). At doses of 0.3 and 1 μg, EGF promoted little angiogenesis, whereas TGF-α triggered extensive formation of new capillaries. At the 10-μg dose, EGF also induced extensive angiogenesis. Histological examination showed that there was no inflammatory response after the administration of either growth factor (Schreiber et al. 1986).

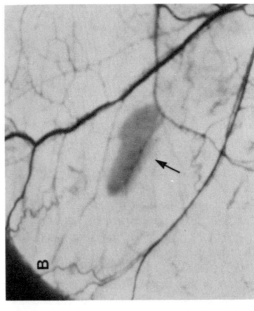

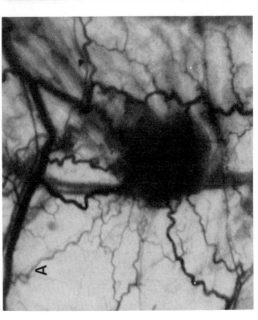

Figure 1 Angiogenic stimulation by TGF-α and EGF in the hamster cheek pouch in vivo 5 days after subcutaneous injection of 1 μg of TGF-α (A) and 1 μg of EGF (B) adsorbed on agarose beads. Note the absence of angiogenesis in B around the agarose beads (arrow) and the tortuosity of vessels in A. For the angiogenesis assay, male Syrian golden hamsters of the same age were anesthetized. The left cheek pouch was everted, and mitogens, dissolved in 10 μl of sterile saline and then adsorbed into 10 μl of Cibachrome blue agarose, were injected subcutaneously. Five days later, the animals were again anesthetized, and the extent of neovascularization in the pouch was evaluated. Magnification, 4 ×.

74

In conclusion, our data indicate that TGF-α and EGF bind equally effectively to the EGF receptors on several cell types, including endothelial cells, and appear to be equally potent mitogens in vitro for endothelial cells. It was reported previously that EGF has angiogenic activity (Gospodarowicz et al. 1979) and can induce a mitogenic response in microvascular endothelial cells (McAuslan et al. 1985). Our data indicate that, in vivo, TGF-α is more effective than EGF in promoting angiogenesis. It is unfortunately very difficult to quantitate accurately the differences between the angiogenesis induced by TGF-α and that induced by EGF because of the complexity of the morphological appearance of the neovascularization pattern. These quantitative differences in activity could conceivably be due to a lower sensitivity of TGF-α to protease digestion in vivo, to differences in clearance ratios, or to other factors that would result in a higher bioavailability of TGF-α. However, the two peptides had similar kinetics of release, and they were previously found to be equipotent in an eyelid-opening assay in newborn mice, suggesting that they have similar pharmacological properties (Smith et al. 1985). It is also possible that, in addition to binding to the EGF receptor, TGF-α binds to another receptor that plays a role in the promotion of angiogenesis. There could be high- and low-affinity EGF receptors, as suggested by, for example, Gregoriou and Rees (1984), and these might display different binding parameters for EGF and TGF-α. Even if we assume that there is only one type of EGF receptor, we might postulate that TGF-α and EGF interact differently with the receptor at the cell surface or during internalization of the ligand-receptor complex. Another possibility is that, in vivo, both growth factors induce the production of angiogenic mediators from another cell type, e.g., fibroblasts, in addition to the endothelial cells. If this were the case, these cells would have to display a differential response to TGF-α and EGF. Differences in potency between TGF-α and EGF have also been observed in the ability to induce bone formation (Stern et al. 1985; Ibbotson et al. 1986) and keratinocyte colony formation (Y. Barrandon and H. Green, pers. comm.).

TGF-α: A Possible Role in Tumor Angiogenesis

The relative potency of TGF-α as an angiogenic mediator suggests that, in addition to its potential importance as an autocrine growth regulator, it may play a role in malignancy-associated neovascularization, contributing to the generation of a local microenvironment that is favorable for the growth of solid tumors. This possibility is supported by the observation that TGF-α mRNA cannot be detected in hematopoietic tumor cell lines but is expressed in many solid tumors that undergo neovascularization (Derynck et al. 1987). It is likely that TGF-α functions in a cooperative fashion with other factors or via the induction of the release of angiogenic factors. This assumption is based on the fact that the equal mitogenic effects of TGF-α and EGF on the endothelial cells in vitro cannot explain the differences in angiogenic potencies in vivo. A role for TGF-α in angiogenesis does not exclude the likelihood of other angiogenic mediators secreted by the tumor cells. Several other factors have indeed been shown to be angiogenic factors in various assay systems. Much attention has been focused on basic and acidic fibroblast growth factors, which are potent mitogens for endothelial cells and inducers of neovascularization. Acidic fibroblast growth factor has also been tested in the same hamster cheek pouch systems and induces angiogenesis in a concentration range similar to that of TGF-α (K. Thomas and A. Schreiber, unpubl.). It is thus possible that TGF-α could cooperate with other angiogenic mediators, such as the fibroblast growth factors, in the formation and establishment of the tumor-induced neovascularization.

REFERENCES

Anzano, M.A., A.B. Roberts, C.A. Meyers, A. Komoriya, L.C. Lamb, J.M. Smith, and M.B. Sporn. 1982. Synergistic interaction of two classes of transforming growth factors from murine sarcoma cells. *Cancer Res.* 42: 4776.

De Larco, J.E. and G.J. Todaro. 1978. Growth factors from murine sarcoma virus transformed cells. *Proc. Natl. Acad. Sci.* 75: 4001.

Derynck, R., A.B. Roberts, M.E. Winkler, E.Y. Chen, and D.V. Goeddel. 1984. Human transforming growth factor-α: Precursor structure and expression in *E. coli. Cell* 38: 287.

Derynck, R., D.V. Goeddel, A. Ullrich, J.U. Gutterman, R.D. Williams, T.S. Bringman, and W.H. Berger. 1987. Synthesis of mRNAs for transforming growth factors-α and -β and the epidermal growth factor receptor by human tumors. *Cancer Res.* 47: 707.

Gospodarowicz, D., H. Bialecki, and G.K. Thakral. 1979. The angiogenic activity of fibroblast and epidermal growth factor. *Exp. Eye Res.* 28: 501.

Gregoriou, M. and A.R. Rees. 1984. Properties of a monoclonal antibody to epidermal growth factor receptor with implications for the mechanism of action of EGF. *EMBO J.* 3: 929.

Ibbotson, K.J., J. Harrod, M. Gowen, S. D'Souza, M.E. Winkler, R. Derynck, and G.R. Mundy. 1986. Human recombinant transforming growth factor-α stimulates bone resorption and inhibits formation *in vitro. Proc. Natl. Acad. Sci.* 83: 2228.

Lee, D.C., R.M. Rochford, G.J. Todaro, and L.P. Villareal. 1985. Developmental expression of rat transforming growth factor-α mRNA. *Mol. Cell. Biol.* 5: 3644.

Marquardt, H., M.W. Hunkapiller, L.E. Hood, and G.J. Todaro. 1984. Rat transforming growth factor type 1: Structure and relation to epidermal growth factor. *Science* 223: 1079.

Massagué, J. 1983. Epidermal growth factor-like transforming growth factor. I. Isolation, chemical characterization and potentiation by other transforming growth factors from feline sarcoma virus-transformed rat cells. *J. Biol. Chem.* **258**: 13606.

McAuslan, B.R., V. Bender, W. Riley, and B.A. Moss. 1985. New functions of epidermal growth factor. Stimulation of capillary endothelial cell migration and matrix-dependent proliferation. *Cell. Biol. Int. Rep.* **9**: 175.

Schreiber, A.B., M.E. Winkler, and R. Derynck. 1986. Transforming growth factor-α: A more potent angiogenic mediator than epidermal growth factor. *Science* **232**: 1250.

Smith, M., M.B. Sporn, A.B. Roberts, R. Derynck, M.E. Winkler, and H. Gregory. 1985. Human transforming growth factor-α cause precocious eyelid opening in newborn mice. *Nature* **315**: 515.

Sporn, M.B. and G.J. Todaro. 1980. Autocrine secretion and malignant transformation. *N. Engl. J. Med.* **303**: 878.

Stern, P.H., N.S. Krieger, R.A. Nissenson, R.D. Williams, M.E. Winkler, R. Derynck, and G.J. Strewler. 1985. Human transforming growth factor-α stimulates bone resorption *in vitro*. *J. Clin. Invest.* **76**: 2016.

Todaro, G.J., D.C. Lee, N.R. Webb, T.M. Rose, and J.P. Brown. 1985. Rat type-α transforming growth factor: Structure and possible function as a membrane receptor. In *Cancer cells 3* (ed. J. Feramisco et al.), p. 51. Cold Spring Harbor Laboratory, Cold Spring Harbor, New York.

Winkler, M.E., T.S. Bringman, and B.J. Marks. 1986. The purification of fully active recombinant transforming growth factor-α produced in *Escherichia coli. J. Biol. Chem.* **61**: 13838.

Nonpeptide Angiogenesis Factors

C.C. Haudenschild and M.I. Klibaner

Boston University School of Medicine
Mallory Institute of Pathology
Boston, Massachusetts 02118

Angiogenic activity can be found in samples from almost any class of substances aside from peptides, including lipids, metals, polysaccharides, and synthetic compounds. Many of these compounds initiate or promote the growth of nonvascular cells as well; some (e.g., heparin) may modify the effect of other agents without being growth factors themselves. With few exceptions, nonpeptide factors tend to act indirectly, being part of a cascade of reactions which ultimately result in vascular proliferation. In contrast to some of the growth-promoting peptides and their receptors, which are well-defined molecules, most other factors are still at the stages of isolation, purification, and characterization of specificity. Observation of angiogenic effects under pathophysiological conditions in vivo has often led to the discovery and isolation of such factors, as, for example, in the case of omentum-derived angiogenic lipids.

Revascularization of tissue by the greater omentum was first described by DeRenzi and Boeri (1903); practical surgical applications of the angiogenic properties of attached and isolated omentum as a graft have since been reported by a number of authors. When N. Catsimpoolas learned about the extensive work on omental transposition and grafting by H. Goldsmith, he decided to isolate the active principle. An omental chloroform-methanol extract was found to be angiogenic in the rabbit cornea (Goldsmith et al. 1984). The extract improved collateral perfusion in cat hind legs when injected either locally or at a distant site (Goldsmith et al. 1986). Angiogenic activities were also reported in preparations from cardiac lipids (Silverman et al. 1985) and from differentiated adipocytes in culture (Castellot et al. 1982). Further purification and a systematic evaluation of omentum-derived and other lipids for angiogenic potential are now being performed. This report deals with the use and the interpretation of the chicken CAM (Auerbach et al. 1974) for the evaluation of possible mechanisms for lipid-induced angiogenesis and their relationship to inflammatory processes.

The chicken CAM has large interstitial vessels (Fig. 1A) and a sinusoidal mesh of capillaries (Fig. 1B). The superficial, intraepithelial location of these capillaries is used for gas exchange in the mature

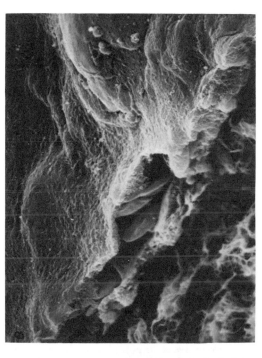

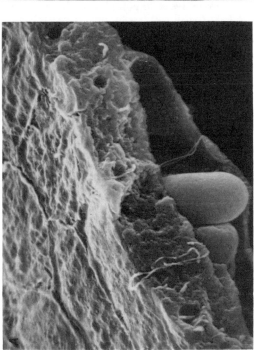

Figure 1 (A) Scanning electron micrograph of an immature chorioallantoic membrane showing an interstitial vessel containing an erythrocyte. (B) Scanning electron micrograph of a mature chorioallantoic membrane showing the intradermal capillaries filled with erythrocytes. Magnifications: (A) 2610 × ; (B) 1740 × .

CAM. The diffusion distance is relatively short for angiogenic factors placed onto the surface of the membrane in an experimental setting. However, the reading of the CAM after 2–3 days for a positive angiogenic reaction is based on the gross morphology of the interstitial vessels which enlarge, show directional growth, and exhibit the typical radial appearance (Fig. 2A). The visibility of the nearby intraepithelial capillaries may be enhanced (Fig. 2B), but this finding reflects predominantly hyperemia or hyperperfusion and can be a transient response to a variety of stimuli. In view of unknown rates of release, resorption, access, or targets of the stimuli, the most simple CAM interpretation appears to be most appropriate for a preliminary screening: the number of negatives after 2 days in multiple sets of 12 readable tests. An approximation of a dose-effect relation can be obtained by subsequent repeats of the tests with different amounts of stimulating factors. For further evaluation of the specificity of the response and the nature of possible angiogenic mechanisms, we refer to histological examination and to tests in different vascular beds of other species.

From our experience with this approach, we can propose a number of mechanisms by which omental and other lipids (which may be quite inert by themselves) may have angiogenic effects. One of these mechanisms may be recognized as a "focal substrate overload" for enzyme reactions that result in active compounds, such as certain known angiogenic prostanoids (Form and Auerbach 1983). For example, 10 μg of arachidonic acid consistently elicits a response of zero to one negative out of 12 tests. Similar amounts of eicosapentaenoic acid did not show this effect.

A second mechanism, which might take place, for example, with fatty acids, could consist of changes in the fluidity of the cell membranes, especially when these molecules accumulate temporarily in free form, acting as detergents. Such detergent mechanisms may mimic strong, albeit nonspecific, growth signals in situations where protective fatty-acid-binding mechanisms are temporarily and locally overwhelmed. The effects of different fatty acids are variable; oleic acid in picogram amounts can stimulate the CAM, whereas linoleic acid is less effective. Large local doses of oleic acid are outright cytotoxic and inflammatory, and the vascularity appearing at such sites represents the vascular part of a tissue response to a chemical burn, i.e., one or several indirect angiogenic mechanisms.

Qualitatively, CAM inflammation consistently exhibits a strong angiogenic component, whereas the infiltrative and nonvascular proliferative components vary widely. Figure 3A shows an extensive, acute inflammatory response: Vascular manifestations are the increase in number, size, and filling of vascular profiles; edema is a sign of per-

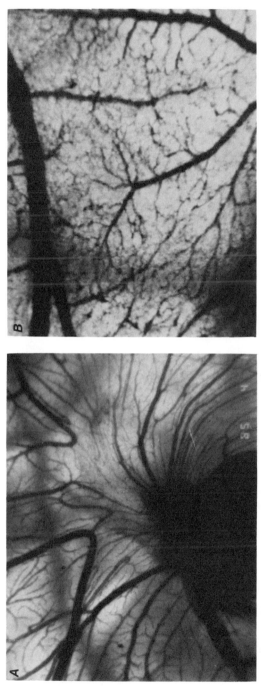

Figure 2 (A) Positive CAM reaction; large vessel loops point toward the disk of boiled egg shell membrane containing oleic acid. (B) Hyperemia of intraepithelial capillaries enhances their visibility.

81

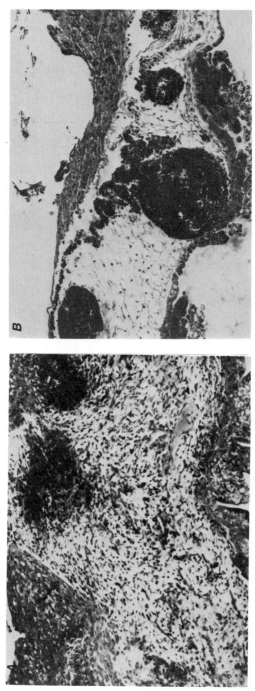

Figure 3 (A) CAM response with all inflammatory components present: increased number and size of blood vessels, ecto-, endo-, and mesodermal proliferation, as well as edema and inflammatory cell infiltrate. (B) Selective response: enlargement and overfilling of blood vessels, proliferative ecto- and endodermal response, but absence of mesenchymal fibroblast proliferation and absence of inflammatory cell infiltrate. Magnifications: (A) 139 ×; (B) 139 ×.

82

meability change. Nonvascular proliferation is seen in all three embryonic layers (mesenchymal fibroblasts and ecto- and endodermal epithelia), and the cellularity is further increased by massive infiltration with polymorpho- and mononuclear inflammatory cells. In contrast, in Figure 3B, these inflammatory infiltrates are absent and mesenchymal proliferation is limited to very prominent blood vessels; what prevents this specimen from representing entirely pure, noninflammatory angiogenesis is the marked proliferation of both ecto- and endodermal epithelia. With thorough histological examination, it is indeed very difficult to find marked blood vessel growth in the absence of any other infiltrative or proliferative response, even in hydrocortisone-treated CAMs. Distinction between angiogenesis per se and inflammatory response with a marked, predominant vascular component is difficult; the extent and nature of the nonvascular components of the response may vary and may need to be evaluated separately.

Finally, complex lipids may act indirectly, typically by causing locally accumulated factors to be released, or by temporarily changing the sensitivity of migrating or blood-borne cells to stimuli that cause them to slow down, adhere, and release their own mitogens. Highly purified complex lipids can be completely inert; yet when presented to the mediating cell in combination with a carrier that may be equally inert by itself, cell activation may occur and may cause angiogenesis (Gullino 1986), even at a distant site. Likely targets are sites where signals for cellular infiltration and release of growth factors are already at an elevated level, such as in wounds or near necrotic areas. Tissues characterized by unusually rapid cell disintegration (this could include blood clots) can thus become a source, as well as a target, of lipid and other angiogenic factors. In the absence of such targets, lipid-mediated activation may have no effect at all. Although many of these mechanisms are still speculative, the recognition of certain lipids as a distinct class of nonpeptide angiogenic factors can stimulate future research along these hypotheses.

ACKNOWLEDGMENT
This work has been supported by Angio-Medical Corp. (president: R.S. Sinn).

REFERENCES
Auerbach, R., L. Kubai, D. Knighton, and J. Folkman. 1974. A simple procedure for the long-term cultivation of chicken embryos. *Dev. Biol.* **41**: 391.

Castellot, J.J., Jr., M.J. Karnovsky, and B.M. Spiegelman. 1982. Differentiation-dependent stimulation of neovascularization and endothelial cell chemotaxis by 3T3 adipocytes. *Proc. Natl. Acad. Sci.* **79**: 5597.

DeRenzi, E. and G. Boeri. 1903. Das Netz als ein Schutzorgan. *Berl. Klin. Wchschr.* **40**: 773.

Form, D.M. and R. Auerbach. 1983. PGE2 and angiogenesis. *Proc. Soc. Exp. Biol. Med.* **172**: 214.

Goldsmith, H.S., A.L. Griffith, and N. Catsimpoolas. 1986. Increased vascular perfusion after administration of an omental lipid fraction. *Surgery* **162**: 578.

Goldsmith, H.S., A.L. Griffith, A. Kupferman, and N. Catsimpoolas. 1984. Lipid angiogenic factor from omentum. *J. Am. Med. Assoc.* **252**: 2034.

Gullino, P. 1986. Considerations on the mechanisms of the angiogenic response. *Anticancer Res.* **6**: 153.

Silverman, K.J., D.P. Lund, B.R. Zetter, L.L. Lainey, J.A. Shahood, D.G. Freiman, J. Folkman, and C. Barger. 1985. Fat angiogenesis: A possible link to coronary atherosclerosis and thrombosis. *Circulation* (supple. III) **72**: 282.

Differentiation-dependent Stimulation of Angiogenesis by 3T3-Adipocytes

J.J. Castellot, Jr.* and B.M. Spiegelman[†]

*Department of Pathology, Harvard Medical School
and [†]Dana-Farber Cancer Institute, Boston, Massachusetts 02115

Adipocyte differentiation and angiogenesis are tightly coordinated during embryological development. We therefore tested the ability of adipocyte-conditioned medium to stimulate neovascularization in vivo (Castellot et al. 1982). Conditioned medium from 3T3-adipocytes stimulated new blood vessel growth in the chick chorioallantoic membrane (CAM). Control (unconditioned) medium or conditioned medium from preadipocytes did not stimulate neovascularization, even at much higher doses. Thus, the production of the angiogenic activity was strongly dependent on differentiation of the adipocytes.

Because neovascularization appears to involve the activation of endothelial cell protease activity, chemotaxis, and mitogenesis, we tested the ability of 3T3-adipocytes to stimulate these endothelial cell activities in vitro (Castellot et al. 1980, 1982, 1986). Adipocyte-conditioned medium strongly stimulated protease activity, chemotaxis, and proliferation of endothelial cells. 3T3-preadipocytes produced < 10% as much of these activities as 3T3-adipocytes, indicating that these in vitro activities are also strongly differentiation-dependent. The mitogenic and chemotactic activities were specific for vascular endothelial cells in that no other cell type examined was stimulated by adipocyte-conditioned medium.

Temporal Correlation of Differentiation and Production of Angiogenic Activities

To examine the relationship between differentiation and secretion of angiogenic activities by 3T3-adipocytes, we carried out a time course of production of angiogenic and chemotactic activities. The data indicate that secretion of this activity is a very early event, detectable within 3 days after the cells become confluent, and is concomitant with lipogenesis and induction of the differentiation-specific lipogenic enzymes. It is independent of the amount of lipid the cell has accumulated, since the activity remains constant even as the amount of intracellular lipid is rapidly increasing from day 3 to day 14. This further supports the hypothesis that angiogenesis and differentiation are tightly coupled events.

Pharmacological Studies

Because adipocytes have been shown to synthesize prostaglandins (Negrel and Ailhaud 1981), and because prostaglandins have been reported to stimulate neovascularization in vivo (Ben-Ezra 1978; Ziche et al. 1982; Form and Auerbach 1983), we treated adipocytes with indomethacin during the conditioning period. When conditioned medium from indomethacin-treated adipocytes was tested for its ability to stimulate neovascularization in vivo and endothelial cell proliferation and chemotaxis in vitro, a marked reduction in all of these activities was seen. In addition, the dose response of the indomethacin effect on adipocytes indicated that this agent was effective at doses considered to specifically inhibit the cyclooxygenase pathway ($ED_{50} = 1 \times 10^{-7}$M). To reduce the possibility of a non-cyclooxygenase-mediated effect of indomethacin, we also tested the ability of another cyclooxygenase inhibitor, ibuprofen, to block the angiogenic activities, and virtually identical results were obtained. The possibility that indomethacin blocked production of angiogenic activities by adversely affecting differentiation is very unlikely, since levels of drug which inhibit secretion of angiogenic activities do not interfere with lipogenesis or with differentiation-dependent protein biosynthesis. These data suggest that a fatty acid cyclooxygenase product is on the biosynthetic pathway for the angiogenic factors, is a cofactor required for the angiogenic molecule(s), or is operating indirectly by affecting the processing or secretion of other angiogenic molecules by adipocytes.

Fractionation and Identification

The angiogenic activity is extracted from conditioned medium into organic solvents. In light of this, we fractionated adipocyte-conditioned medium by reversed-phase chromatography on C-18 columns. Both the angiogenesis- and chemotaxis-stimulating activities eluted at 30–50% ethanol, a profile also obtained for authentic prostanoid standards. Interestingly, the mitogenic activity eluted with the aqueous flow-through, and little or no mitogenic activity eluted with ethanol, indicating that the stimulation of angiogenesis is a multicomponent process.

Further fractionation of the angiogenic activities was carried out by pooling the 30–50% ethanol fractions from the C-18 column and subjecting them to thin-layer chromatography, using buffer systems for separating arachidonate metabolites (Salmon and Flower 1982). The data demonstrate that there are at least two distinct lipophilic components that stimulate angiogenesis and chemotaxis activities. One of the fractions, which accounts for approximately 10–20% of the total angiogenic activity, comigrated with authentic prostaglandins E_1 and E_2 (PGE_1 and PGE_2). When this fraction was extracted with ethanol and rechromatographed in a different buffer system, the angiogenic activity again comigrated with PGE_1 and PGE_2 standards. We have thus tentatively concluded that one of the angiogenic activities is a member of the PGE family.

Corroboration for this comes from three sources. First, when authentic PGE_1 and PGE_2 were tested in the angiogenesis assay, both were found to be active at the levels secreted by adipocytes. Other PGs, including PGF_{1a}, PGF_{2a}, and 6-keto-F_{1a} (the major metabolite of prostacyclin, PGI_2), required at least 100-fold higher concentrations. The angiogenic ability of PGEs confirms the results of other laboratories mentioned above. Second, indomethacin treatment of the adipocytes during the conditioning period eliminated $> 90\%$ of the activity in this fraction, confirming the presence of a cyclooxygenase product. Third, radioimmunoassay for PGE_1 and PGE_2 in adipocyte-conditioned medium revealed that PGE_1 was present at approximately 2 ng/ml and PGE_2 was present at about 13 ng/ml, indicating that the adipocytes are secreting significant quantities of PGEs under our culture conditions. The synthesis of PGEs is only slightly differentiation-dependent (less than twofold), as measured by radioimmunoassay of adipocyte- and preadipocyte-secreted material.

The second active fraction, which we have designated TLC5, accounts for approximately 80–90% of the adipocyte-secreted angiogenic activity and is almost totally differentiation-dependent. It does not comigrate with any of the 13 prostanoid or other standards we have used, including prostaglandins A_2, B_2, D_2, E_1, E_2, F_{1a}, F_{2a}, 6-keto-F_{1a}, 15-keto-E_2, 13,14-dihydro-15-keto-E_2, 15-keto-F_{2a}, 13,14-dihydro-15-keto-F_{2a}, thromboxane B_2, arachidonate, oleate, adenosine, and thymidine. TLC5 also possesses significantly more chemoattractant capacity than the PGE fraction, accounting for approximately 80% of the starting activity. Its organic solubility and chromatographic properties suggest that TLC5 may be an unusual or even a novel polar lipid.

In summary, the fractionation experiments have clearly demonstrated that (1) multiple endothelial-cell-stimulating signals are produced by adipocytes, since mitogenic factors and chemotactic factors can be distinguished; (2) the mitogen is not angiogenic at its normally secreted concentration, whereas the two lipophilic factors stimulate both angiogenesis and chemotaxis; and (3) one of the lipophilic factors appears to be E-series prostaglandins; the other lipophilic component is very potent, strongly differentiation-dependent, and may be an unusual or novel polar lipid.

Effect of Heparin on Angiogenesis

We had observed that the addition of heparin to adipocyte-conditioned medium potentiated the angiogenic response, but heparin itself had no effect when tested in the CAM assay (Castellot et al. 1982). This observation was similar to that made by Taylor and Folkman (1982), who found that heparin potentiated the angiogenic response to tumor extracts. We have examined the cellular mechanisms by which heparin potentiates the ability of 3T3-adipocytes to stimulate the formation of new blood vessels (Castellot et al. 1986). Both anticoagulant and nonanticoagulant heparin species enhanced the angiogenic activity of adipocyte-secreted products in the CAM assay, indicating that the angiotropic effect of this glycosaminoglycan is independent of its effect on the coagulation cascade. Other glycosaminoglycans were unable to potentiate angiogenesis. We examined the ability of heparin to modulate in vitro the following three endothelial functions thought to be related to angiogenesis: protease activity, motility, and mitogenesis. Heparin caused a 100% increase in the adipocyte-induced stimulation of endothelial cell plasminogen activator (PA) activity and motility but had no effect on proliferation. The enhancement of PA and chemoattractant activities had a similar ED_{50} (1–2 μg/ml) and optimum dose (10–30 μg/ml).

When we examined the direct effect of heparin on the activities of two distinct PA enzymes—urokinase and tissue type—a dual action of heparin was observed: tissue-type enzyme activity was stimulated 100% by heparin at 10 μg/ml, whereas urokinase activity was inhibited by 77% at this dose. These data suggest that heparin potentiates angiogenesis in vivo by stimulating endothelial cell PA, motility, or both. Our results further suggest that for adipocyte-induced blood vessel formation, in contrast to other angiogenesis systems, heparin does not appear to affect the mitogenic activity.

REFERENCES

Ben-Ezra, D. 1978. Neovascularization of prostaglandins, growth factors, and synthetic chemoattractants. *Amer. J. Ophthalmol.* **86**: 455.

Castellot, J.J., M.J. Karnovsky, and B.M. Spiegelman. 1980. Potent stimulation of vascular endothelial cell growth by differentiated 3T3 adipocytes. *Proc. Natl. Acad. Sci.* **77**: 6007.

———. 1982. Differentiation-dependent stimulation of neovascularization and endothelial cell chemotaxis by 3T3 adipocytes. *Proc. Natl. Acad. Sci.* **79**: 5597.

Castellot, J.J., A.M. Kambe, D.E. Dobson, and B.M. Spiegelman. 1986. Heparin potentiation of 3T3-adipocyte stimulated angiogenesis: Mechanisms of action on endothelial cells. *J. Cell. Physiol.* **127**: 323.

Form, D. and R. Auerbach. 1983. PGE_2 and angiogenesis. *Proc. Soc. Exp. Biol. Med.* **172**: 214.

Negrel, R. and G. Ailhaud. 1981. Metabolism of arachidonic acid and prostaglandin synthesis in the preadipocyte clonal line of OB_{17}. *Biochem. Biophys. Res. Commun.* **98**: 768.

Salmon, J.A. and R.J. Flower. 1982. Extraction and thin-layer chromatograpy of arachidonic acid metabolites. *Methods Enzymol.* **86**: 477.

Taylor, S. and J. Folkman. 1982. Protamine is an inhibitor of angiogenesis. *Nature* **297**: 307.

Ziche, M., J. Jones, and P. Gullino. 1982. Role of PGE_1 and copper in angiogenesis. *J. Natl. Cancer Inst.* **69**: 475.

Hyaluronic Acid and Its Degradation Products Modulate Angiogenesis In Vivo and In Vitro

S. Kumar and D. West

Christie Hospital and Holt Radium Institute
Manchester, M20 9BX, England

Native hyaluronic acid (HA) and its degradation products have profound effects on endothelial cells in vivo and in vitro.

The extracellular matrix (ECM), which is ubiquitously present around cells in vivo, is no longer considered an inert space-filler. On the contrary, the ECM is thought to influence the geometry, metabolism, and gene expression of cells via transmembrane receptors and the cytoskeleton, which in turn controls ECM synthesis. HA is a major component of the ECM and was first described in mammalian tissues in 1934. It is a negatively charged, high-molecular-weight glycosaminoglycan (GAG) consisting of repeating disaccharide units of N-acetylglucosamine and glucuronate. It differs from other GAGs in its lack of sulfation and absence of covalently linked protein. HA has been reported to have a role in embryogenesis, tissue healing, and numerous pathological states in adult life. For instance, during embryonic differentiation and wound healing, HA levels are initially high and then decrease rapidly in response to an increase in hyaluronidase (HAase). Furthermore, the molecular size of HA fragments can vary during the course of embryogenesis and tissue repair (Toole et al. 1986).

HA and Angiogenesis

Regarding the role of HA in angiogenesis, undoubtedly there are many gaps in our knowledge of HA in endothelial cell function, but a considerable number of important facts are known. Under pathological conditions associated with abnormal angiogenesis, such as tumors, diabetic retinopathy, and rheumatoid arthritis, neovascularization occurs adjacent to a hyaluronate-rich fluid or stroma. Elevated levels of circulating HA are seen in the sera of patients with cancer, rheumatoid arthritis, and psoriasis. This suggests that freely diffusible and degraded HA is produced at these sites of vessel formation. This is supported by observations that tissue-cultured rheumatoid synovial cells and activated synovial fibroblasts synthesize increased amounts of

HA that has a much lower molecular weight than that produced by normal cells. Histochemical studies have demonstrated that the GAGs of mature vessels differ from those of newly formed capillary sprouts. At the migrating tip of a capillary sprout, the basal lamina contains mainly HA, which perhaps aids endothelial cell migration and serves as a substrate for the mature lamina.

The present study resulted from our initial observations that the unfractionated human wound fluid was not angiogenic on the chick chorioallantoic membrane (CAM), but after purification it induced an angiogenic response. Recombination experiments gave a strong indication that wound fluid contains both angiogenic and antiangiogenic components. We postulated that the inhibitory component of wound fluid was HA; therefore, wound fluid was digested with HAase. After HAase treatment, the wound fluids induced a very potent angiogenic reaction in the CAM assay. Further work involved the treatment of native HA with HAase, and it was quickly and firmly established that (1) completely degraded HA has no effect on angiogenesis and (2) only HA fragments of a certain molecular size were capable of inducing angiogenesis (West et al. 1985b).

Oligosaccharides of HA and Angiogenesis

Three different HAs (human umbilical vein, bovine vitreous, and HA provided by Fermatech) were digested with bovine testicular hyaluronidase for various time intervals with the following results. Digests of HA obtained within a period of 1–10 hours were consistently positive on the CAM, compared with undigested HA or HA digested for 24 hours or longer ($p < 0.0003$, χ^2-test). A precise estimate of the size was obtained using (1) column chromatography with Sephadex G-50 (superfine) 200×2.5 cm and (2) polyacrylamide gel electrophoresis (PAGE). When the data were analyzed, taking into consideration possible overlap between fractions, it was concluded that the only HA fragments to be angiogenic were those in the 4- to 16-disaccharide range. The minimum amount of fragments required to induce an angiogenic response in a CAM assay was found to be 1 μg.

In vitro studies were carried out to examine the effects of HA and its fragments on tissue-cultured bovine brain capillary and aortic endothelial cells.

HA and Endothelial Cell Proliferation In Vitro

Bovine capillary and aortic endothelial cells were cultured in 24-well plates, at 10^4 cells/well, and allowed to adhere overnight. The cells were then incubated in 0.5 ml of medium containing 0.1–100 μg of HA oligosaccharides with or without [^{3}H]TdR. After 72 hours, the wells were washed and either cells were harvested to determine the uptake of radioactivity or the adherent cell number was measured by fluorimetric estimation of cellular DNA (West et al. 1985a). The minimal amount of HA fragments that produced a statistically significant enhancement of the uptake of [³H]thymidine or resulted in an increase in cell numbers was between 0.5 and 1.0 μg/ml (Fig. 1). The greatest stimulation was given by those HA oligomers (F3) which were the most angiogenic in the CAM assay.

HA and Endothelial Cell Migration
Migration studies were performed in 13-mm Swinnex filter units (Millipore) fitted with a 12-μm pore-size filter. Bovine aortic endothelial cells (10^5 cells/filter) were introduced into the top chamber, and the bottom chamber was filled with different concentrations of HA fragments in the same medium. Migration was allowed to proceed for 18 hours, after which the filters were removed, fixed, and stained, and migration was measured using a microscope fitted with a vernier calibration scale. The results were expressed relative to the control using medium alone. The maximal value for migration induced by HA fragments was 149% of control ($p < 0.05$).

HA Binds to Endothelial Cells
In a preliminary study, bovine aortic endothelial cells incubated for 60 minutes in a tissue-culture medium containing HA fragments, followed by extensive washing, proliferated more than control untreated cells. These experiments showed that HA fragments can bind to endothelial cells.

Native HA and Its Fragments and the
Endothelial Cell Monolayer
Confluent monolayers of endothelial cells showed little change in morphology after 4 hours in the presence of either native HA or its fragments. After 24 hours, the effect of HA was dependent on its size. Native HA inhibited proliferation at low concentrations, and at higher concentrations it disrupted the endothelial cell monolayer. The latter was not an irreversible cytotoxic effect, as a cobblestone monolayer reformed when HA was removed.

HA and Endothelial Cell Membrane
Using an electron spin resonance technique, it was found that HA fragments increased the fluidity of endothelial cell membranes.

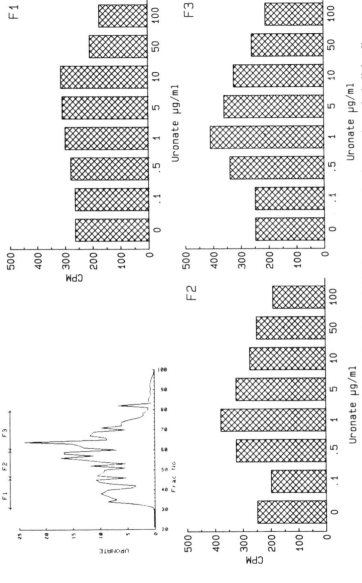

Figure 1 Effect of fractionated HA fragments on bovine aortic endothelial cells.

CONCLUSION

The most significant finding of the present study is that HA fragments (4–16 disaccharides long) induce angiogenesis in vivo and stimulate proliferation and migration of endothelial cells in vitro. In contrast, high concentrations of native HA inhibit the proliferation of endothelial cells and disrupt monolayers. HA fragments bind to endothelial cells; furthermore, the addition of HA fragments to isolated endothelial cell membranes increases the membrane fluidity. Clearly, further studies using in vitro models will allow us to understand the mode of action of native HA and its oligosaccharides, which in turn may lead to modulation of angiogenesis in situations where it is deficient or excessive (Kumar and Arnold 1986). Since HA is readily obtainable from natural sources, it might prove easy to manipulate its concentration in these tissues.

REFERENCES

Kumar, S. and F. Arnold. 1986. Can metastasis be restrained in breast cancer? In: *Breast cancer: Treatment and prognosis* (ed. B.A. Stoll), p. 287. Blackwell Scientific Publications, England.

Toole, B.P., C.B. Knudson, W. Knudson, R.L. Goldberg, G. Chi-Rosso, and C. Biswas. 1986. In *Mesenchymal-epithelial interactions in neural development* (ed. T.R. Wolff). Springer-Verlag, Berlin. (In press.)

West, D.C., A. Sattar, and S. Kumar. 1985a. A simplified in situ solubilization procedure for the determination of DNA and cell number in tissue cultured mammalian cells. *Anal. Biochem.* **147**: 289.

West, D.C., I.N. Hampson, F. Arnold, and S. Kumar. 1985b. Angiogenesis induced by degradation products of hyaluronic acid. *Science* **228**: 1324.

Inhibitors of Angiogenesis: Angiostatic Steroids

J. Folkman*[†] and D.E. Ingber*[†‡]

*Department of Surgery, Children's Hospital, Boston, Massachusetts 02115
*[†]Department of Surgery, Anatomy, and Cellular Biology and [‡]Department of Pathology, Harvard Medical School, Boston, Massachusetts 02115

Within the past 2 years, at least four different angiogenic peptides have been reported for which the protein sequence and gene structure are now known: (1) heparin-binding growth factors (which include endothelial cell growth factor and acidic and basic fibroblast growth factors) (Shing et al. 1984; Esch et al. 1985; Thomas et al. 1985; Jaye et al. 1986); (2) transforming growth factor-α (Schreiber et al. 1986); (3) transforming growth factor-β (Roberts et al. 1986); and (4) angiogenin (Fett et al. 1985; Kurachi et al. 1985; Strydom et al. 1985). The first three are found in many normal tissues as well as in tumors. In fact, the heparin-binding endothelial cell growth factors are so ubiquitous that a useful question may be, Are there any tissues that do not contain them?

The capillary endothelial cells in these tissues are usually quiescent. Unlike muscosal cells of the gut or hematopoietic cells of the bone marrow in which proliferation is so rapid that turnover times are measured in days, the turnover time of vascular endothelial cells is measured in years (Denekamp 1984). With the exception of the brief bursts of physiological angiogenesis that seem to be unique to females (e.g., occurring during ovulation, repair of the menstruating uterus, and placentation), angiogenesis is rarely observed unless it is of pathological origin. Thus, a male may live an entire lifetime without angiogenesis, unless he is wounded or develops a disease dominated by neovascularization.

We can ask, How are vascular endothelial cells normally maintained at such extremely low proliferation rates in the presence of such abundant growth factors? On a theoretical basis, there must be mechanisms that prevent endothelial cells from proliferating under normal conditions but that can be overcome or perhaps down-regulated when neovascularization is required, e.g., during wound healing. We have recently discovered a new class of "angiostatic" steroids that circulate in the plasma and that were previously thought to be biologically inactive metabolites of cortisone (Crum et al. 1985). We propose that these compounds may restrict the growth of capillary endothelial cells and thus represent one example of a normal inhibiting mechanism.

95

This new steroid function was revealed from a series of experiments on the role of heparin in angiogenesis. During a histological study of the various cell types involved in tumor angiogenesis, mast cells were observed to increase about 40-fold at the site of a tumor implant *before* new capillary sprouts converged upon the tumor (Kessler et al. 1976). Mast-cell heparin was found to stimulate locomotion (Zetter 1980) of capillary endothelial cells in vitro (Azizkhan et al. 1980) and to augment tumor angiogenesis in vivo (Taylor and Folkman 1982). Heparin was then used by us (Taylor and Folkman 1982; Shing et al. 1985) and by others (Castellot et al. 1986) to potentiate neovascularization induced by substances being tested for angiogenic activity in the chick embryo. Angiogenesis that only began to appear at 3 days without heparin became visible after only 1 day in the presence of heparin. A complication of using chick chorioallantoic membrane (Folkman and Cotran 1976) was that egg shell dust occasionally fell on the membrane and caused inflammatory neovascularization (which was also potentiated by heparin). Application of cortisone or hydrocortisone to the chorioallantoic membrane prevented the inflammatory reaction but did not interfere with tumor-induced angiogenesis. When heparin and cortisone were applied together, however, tumor angiogenesis was also inhibited. Furthermore, there was regression of growing capillaries in the 6-day chorioallantoic membrane (Folkman et al. 1983). This unexpected synergism was independent of the anticoagulant activity of heparin. In fact, nonanticoagulant hexasaccharide fragments of heparin produced by enzymatic cleavage (Folkman et al. 1983), or synthetic pentasaccharide heparin fragments (Crum et al. 1985), were more potent than whole heparin. The anti-angiogenic activity of heparin-steroid mixtures was unrelated to the anti-inflammatory (glucocorticoid) or salt-retaining (mineralocorticoid) properties of the corticosteroids, because a biologically inactive stereoisomer of hydrocortisone, 11a-hydrocortisone (epicortisol), was equally effective in causing capillary regression in the presence of heparin (Crum et al. 1985).

Angiostatic activity appears to be governed by distinct structural configurations of the pregnane nucleus (Crum et al. 1985). The 11- and 21-hydroxyl groups can be removed without significant loss of angiostatic activity, but removal of the 17-hydroxyl group reduces antiangiogenic activity by about 76% of the activity of hydrocortisone (Crum et al. 1985). Reduction of the "A" ring (e.g., removal of the 4,5, double bond) increases anti-angiogenic activity by about twice that of hydrocortisone. Pregnenolone, a derivative of cholesterol and a precursor for the biosynthesis of the adrenal corticoids, is inactive, as are structures such as progesterone, where the 11-, 17-, and 21-hydroxyl groups are all absent. Tetrahydrocortisol, a natural metabolite of cortisone previously considered to be biologically inactive (Liddle and Melmon 1974), is one of the most potent naturally occurring angiostatic steroids. Synthetic angiostatic steroids exhibit greater anti-angiogenic activity than most of the natural steroids.

To elucidate a mechanism of action for these angiostatic steroids, it is instructive to compare (Ingber et al. 1986) regressing capillary blood vessels with epithelial tissues that undergo involution, e.g., mammary gland (Wicha et al. 1980) and Mullerian duct (Ikawa et al. 1984). In both tissues, involution of epithelium was associated with, or preceded by, breakdown of the basement membrane. Therefore, we used immunofluorescence microscopy to study the distribution of two basement-membrane components, fibronectin and laminin, in growing and regressing capillary blood vessels (Ingber et al. 1986). In normal 6–8-day chorioallantoic membranes, fibronectin and laminin appeared in continuous linear patterns within the basement membrane surrounding growing capillaries. In contrast, chorioallantoic membranes treated with combinations of angiostatic steroid and heparin exhibited capillary basement-membrane fragmentation and eventually complete loss of fibronectin and laminin from regions of capillary involution. Capillary basement-membrane breakdown correlated with capillary retraction, endothelial cell rounding, and associated capillary regression. The basement membranes of surrounding large vessels, neighboring epithelium, and nongrowing capillaries were not affected.

The mechanism by which only the basement membrane of growing capillaries breaks down, leaving the basement membranes of neighboring epithelium and large vessels intact, is not obvious. In normal chorioallantoic membrane, the subectodermal capillary bed undergoes rapid extension in association with continuous basement-membrane accumulation. Various angiogenic factors also stimulate the production of proteases and collagenases by capillary endothelial cells (Gross et al. 1983; Kalebic et al. 1983). Growth and migration of endothelial cells in vitro are similarly associated with both deposition and degradation of basement-membrane components (Madri and Stenn 1982; Kalebic et al. 1983). These observations suggest that high rates of basement-membrane turnover may be required for capillary growth. In contrast, adjacent tissues that do not undergo regression may be relatively more static or formalized structures. Angiostatic steroids do not cause capillary regression when applied to older chorioallantoic membranes that, as previously shown (Ausprunk et al. 1974), contain nongrowing capillaries. These older capillaries are surrounded by a more complete basement membrane (e.g., containing increased amount of laminin and type IV collagen). Therefore, the basement membrane of growing capillaries may be more sensitive to pharmacologic perturbation by angiostatic steroids. This class of steroids also appears to have greater specificity for capillaries than for epithelial tissues.

Capillary basement-membrane dissolution is the first biochemical action identified for this new class of antiangiogenic steroids when they are administered at pharmacological doses. At these doses, the base-ment-membrane alterations induced by the angiostatic steroids could act to regulate the growth and viability of endothelial cells. We have previously presented a model of tissue regulation in which the growth and development of a cell population may be modulated through directed structural alterations in basement membranes that produce changes in cell shape (Ingber and Jamieson 1985). Rounding of capillary endothelial cells could result from changes in the basement membrane, such as release of fibronectin fragments. Normal endothelial cells progressively lose their ability to grow in response to stimulation by angiogenic factors as they take on increasingly rounded forms (D.E. Ingber et al., in prep.), and they do not survive in the unattached (completely spherical) state (Hayman et al. 1985).

Angiostatic steroids, such as tetrahydrocortisol, occur physiologically at low concentrations. It is not clear how these low concentrations could regulate the growth of capillary endothelial cells, especially in the absence of exogenous heparin. However, it is possible that low levels of circulating angiostatic steroids may act synergistically with heparin-like molecules on the endothelial cell surface and in its basement membrane to restrain endothelial cell growth. Experimental proof of this concept remains to be demonstrated.

The discovery of angiostatic steroids indicates that distinct conformations of the steroid molecule convey specificity for growing capillary endothelial cells. The existence of molecules with this biological activity suggests that there may be other naturally occurring inhibitors of capillary endothelial growth that help to maintain vascular endothelial cells in their normal resting state.

REFERENCES

Ausprunk, D.H., D.R. Knighton, and J. Folkman. 1974. Differentiation of vascular endothelium in the chick chorioallantois: A structural and autoradiographic study. *Dev. Biol.* **38**: 237.

Azizkhan, R.G., J.C. Azizkhan, B.R. Zetter, and J. Folkman. 1980. Mast cell heparin stimulates migration of capillary endothelial cells *in vitro*. *J. Exp. Med.* **152**: 931.

Castellot, J.J., Jr., A.M. Kambe, D.E. Dobson, and B.M. Spiegelman. 1986. Heparin potentiation of 3T3-adipocyte stimulated angiogenesis: Mechanisms of action on endothelial cells. *J. Cell. Physiol.* **127**: 323.

Crum, R., S. Szabo, and J. Folkman. 1985. A new class of steroids inhibits angiogenesis in the presence of heparin or a heparin fragment. *Science* **230**: 1375.

Denekamp, J. 1984. Vasculature as a target for tumour therapy. In *Progress in applied microcirculation* (ed. F. Hammersen and O. Hudlicka), p. 28. Karger, Basel.

Esch, F., A. Baird, N. Ling, N. Ueno, F. Hill, L. Denoroy, R. Klepper, D. Gospodarowicz, P. Bohlen, and R. Guillemin. 1985. Primary structure of bovine basic fibroblast growth factor (FGF) and comparison with the amino-terminal sequence of bovine brain acidic FGF. *Proc. Natl. Acad. Sci.* 82: 6507.

Fett, J.W., D.S. Strydom, R.R. Lobb, E.M. Alderman, J.L. Bethune, J.F. Riordan, and B.L. Vallee. 1985. Isolation and characterization of angiogenin, and angiogenic protein from human carcinoma cells. *Biochemistry* 24: 5480.

Folkman, J. and R.S. Cotran. 1976. Relation of vascular proliferation to tumor growth. *Int. Rev. Exp. Pathol.* 16: 207.

Folkman, J., R. Langer, R. Linhardt, C. Haudenschild, and S. Taylor. 1983. Angiogenesis inhibition and tumor regression caused by heparin or a heparin fragment in the presence of cortisone. *Science* 221: 719.

Gross, J.L., D. Moscatelli, and D.B. Rifkin. 1983. Increased capillary endothelial cell protease activity in response to angiogenic stimuli *in vitro*. *Proc. Natl. Acad. Sci.* 80: 2623.

Hayman, E.G., M.D. Pierschenbacher, and E. Ruoslahti. 1985. Detachment of cells from culture substrate by soluble fibronectin peptides. *J. Cell Biol.* 100: 1948.

Ikawa, H., R.L. Trelstad, J.M. Hutson, T.F. Manganaro, and P.K. Donahoe. 1984. Changing patterns of fibronectin, laminin, type VI collagen, and a basement membrane proteoglycan during rat Mullerian duct regression. *Dev. Biol.* 102: 260.

Ingber, D.E. and J.D. Jamieson. 1985. Cells as tensegrity structures: Architectural regulation of histodifferentiation by physical forces transduced over basement membrane. In *Gene expression during normal and malignant differentiation* (ed. L.C. Anderson et al.), p. 13, Academic Press, Orlando.

Ingber, D.E., J.A. Madri, and J. Folkman. 1986. A possible mechanism for inhibition of angiogenesis by angiostatic steroids: Induction of capillary basement membrane dissolution. *Endocrinology* 119: 1768.

Jaye, M., R. Howk, W. Burgess, G.A. Ricca, I.-M. Chiu, M.W. Rivera, S.J. O'Brien, W.S. Modi, T. Maciag, and W.N. Drohan. 1986. Human endothelial cell growth factor: Cloning, nucleotide sequence and chromosome localization. *Science* 233: 545.

Kalebic, T., S. Garbisa, B. Glaser, and L.A. Liotta. 1983. Basement membrane collagen: Degradation by migrating endothelial cells. *Science* 221: 281.

Kessler, D.A., R.S. Langer, N.A. Pless, and J. Folkman. 1976. Mast cells and tumor angiogenesis. *Int. J. Cancer* 18: 703.

Kurachi, K., E.W. Davie, D.J. Strydom, J.F. Riordan, and B.L. Vallee. 1985. Sequence of the cDNA and gene for angiogenin, a human angiogenesis factor. *Biochemistry* 24: 5493.

Liddle, G.W. and K.L. Melmon. 1974. In *Textbook of endocrinology* (ed. R.H. Williams), p. 244. Saunders, Philadelphia.

Madri, J.A. and K.S. Stenn. 1982. Aortic endothelial cell migration. I. Matrix requirements and composition. *Am. J. Pathol.* 106: 180.

Roberts, A.B., M.B. Spron, R.K. Assoian, J.M. Smith, N.S. Roche, L.M.

Wakefield, U.I. Heine, L.A. Liotta, V. Falanga, J.H. Kehrl, and A.S. Fauci. 1986. Transforming growth factor type beta: Rapid induction of fibrosis and angiogenesis in vivo and stimulation of collagen formation in vitro. *Proc. Natl. Acad. Sci.* **83**: 4167.

Schreiber, A.B., M.E. Winkler, and R. Derynck. 1986. Transforming growth factor-alpha: A more potent angiogenic mediator than epidermal growth factor. *Science* **232**: 1250.

Shing, Y., J. Folkman, C. Haudenschild, D. Lund, R. Crum, and M. Klagsbrun. 1985. Angiogenesis is stimulated by a tumor-derived growth factor. *J. Cell. Biochem.* **29**: 275.

Shing, Y., J. Folkman, R. Sullivan, C. Butterfield, J. Murray, and M. Klagsbrun. 1984. Heparin affinity: Purification of a tumor-derived capillary endothelial cell growth factor. *Science* **223**: 1296.

Strydom, D.J., J.W. Fett, R.R. Lobb, E.M. Alderman, J.L. Bethune, J.F. Riordan, and B.L. Vallee. 1985. Amino acid sequence of human tumor derived angiogenin. *Biochemistry* **24**: 5486.

Taylor, S. and J. Folkman. 1982. Protamine is an inhibitor of angiogenesis. *Nature* **297**: 307.

Thomas, K.A., M. Rios-Candelore, G. Gimenez-Gallego, J. DiSalvo, J.C. Bennett, J. Rodkey, and S. Fitzpatrick. 1985. Pure brain derived acidic fibroblast growth factor is a potent angiogenic vascular endothelial cell mitogen with sequence homology to interleukin 1. *Proc. Natl. Acad. Sci.* **82**: 6409.

Wicha, M.S., L.A. Liotta, B.K. Vonderhaar, and W.R. Kidwell. 1980. Effects of inhibition of basement membrane collagen deposition on rat mammary gland development. *Dev. Biol.* **80**: 253.

Zetter, B.R. 1980. Migration of capillary endothelial cells is stimulated by tumour derived factors. *Nature* **285**: 41.

Regulation of Metalloproteinase Activity by Microvascular Endothelial Cells

M.J. Banda, G.S. Herron, G. Murphy,*
and Z. Werb

Laboratory of Radiobiology and Environmental Health
University of California, San Francisco, California 94143
*Strangeways Research Laboratory, Cambridge CB14RN, England

The growth of new blood vessels during angiogenesis is associated with three distinct responses by the microvascular endothelium (Folkman 1984). Capillary endothelial cells, which ultimately form the growing tip of a new capillary sprout, must first degrade the basement membrane surrounding intact capillaries. They must then migrate through the extracellular matrix toward the source of the angiogenic stimulus. Proliferation of cells behind the migrating front and formation of a vascular lumen are major events associated with the final phase (Ausprunk and Folkman 1977; Burger et al. 1983). The induction and arrest of capillary endothelial cell migration during neovascularization and angiogenesis are likely to require precise regulation of the synthesis and degradation of extracellular matrix.

Capillary endothelial cells modulate the synthesis and deposition of specific matrix components according to their phenotype. Monolayer resting cells synthesize a continuous subendothelial membrane rich in type IV collagen (Kramer et al. 1985), and migrating or "sprouting" cells switch their synthetic pattern to types I and III collagen (Sage et al. 1981; Madri and Williams 1983).

The production of proteinases by the capillary endothelium is also regulated. Microvascular cells respond to phorbol diester tumor promoters and angiogenic preparations by increasing the expression of latent collagenase and urokinase-type plasminogen activator activities (Gross et al. 1982, 1983). Capillary cells induced to migrate in response to angiogenic preparations produce a membrane-bound enzyme that degrades type IV collagen (Kalebic et al. 1983).

Previous work characterized two metalloproteinases that are coordinately synthesized as latent proenzymes by synovial fibroblasts in response to tumor promoters and agents that perturb cytoskeletal systems (Aggeler et al. 1984a,b): collagenase, which is activatable to a form capable of degrading interstitial collagens (Stricklin et al. 1977;

101

Gross et al. 1980), and stromelysin, which in its activated form has broad substrate specificity for a number of glycoproteins that constitute basement membranes and interstitial tissues, including proteoglycans, fibronectin, laminin, and type IV collagen (Sellers et al. 1977; Galloway et al. 1983; Chin et al. 1985). In contrast to synovial fibroblasts, stimulated capillary endothelial cells express very low levels of protein-ase activity (Gross ct al. 1982, 1983; Moscatelli et al. 1985).

We summarize the evidence that microvascular endothelial cells synthesize and secrete the metalloproteinases collagenase and strome-lysin at a rate comparable to that of fibroblasts and that the expression of proteolytic activity by these cells is regulated by an endogenous proteinase inhibitor, tissue inhibitor of metalloproteinases (TIMP) (Herron et al. 1986a,b). Data are also presented to show that wound-derived preparations stimulate human microvascular endothelial cells to secrete collagenase and TIMP.

RESULTS
Comparison of Proteinase Activities Secreted by Fibroblasts and Microvascular Endothelial Cells

Rabbit brain microvascular endothelial cells (RBCE cells) and rabbit synovial fibroblasts (RSFs) were stimulated with 50 ng/ml of 12-O-tetradecanoylphorbol-13-acetate (TPA) for up to 48 hours. RBCE cells secreted less than 4% of the activatable collagenase and stromelysin per cell secreted by RSFs (Table 1). Experiments were then done to determine whether this difference in activity was due to a difference in rates of synthesis and secretion of proteinase protein, the inability of RBCE cells to activate the metalloproteinase proenzymes, or the action of a proteinase inhibitor.

Table 1 Collagenase and Stromelysin Activities Present in Conditioned Medium of TPA-treated RBCE Cells and RSFs

Time after TPA addition (hr)	Collagenase (units/10^5 cells)		Stromelysin (units/10^5 cells)	
	RBCE cells	RSFs	RBCE cells	RSFs
8	0	0	0	0
15	0	0.1	0.1	n.d.[a]
24	0	3.4	0.2	3.5
31	0.05	3.8	n.d.	n.d.
48	0.10	4.1	0.7	21.0

RBCE cells and RSFs were treated with 50 ng/ml of TPA in serum-free medium. At the indicated times, conditioned medium was removed and assayed for activatable metalloproteinases.

[a] n.d. indicates not determined.

Comparison of Proteinase Protein Synthesis and Secretion Rates in RBCE Cells and RSFs

RBCE cells and RSFs were compared in continuous labeling experiments in which TPA and [^{35}S]methionine were added simultaneously. Immunoprecipitable procollagenase and prostromelysin were analyzed by SDS-polyacrylamide gel electrophoresis followed by autoradiography. Densitometric scans of the autoradiographs showed a comparable secretion of metalloproteinase proteins from both cell types (Table 2), although the rate for RBCE cells was slower.

Ability of RBCE Cells to Activate Metalloproteinases

Because RBCE cells and RSFs synthesize and secrete similar amounts of metalloproteinase proteins, the ability of the proenzyme protein to be activated was investigated. Medium conditioned by TPA-stimulated RBCE cells was treated with 4-aminophenylmercuric acetate (APMA) to activate procollagenase and prostromelysin and analyzed on gelatin-substrate polyacrylamide electrophoretic gels (Fig. 1). Both procollagenase (M_r=57,000 and 53,000) and prostromelysin (M_r=51,000) had gelatinolytic activity. In addition, activated species of the metalloproteinases at a lower molecular weight were detected.

Regulation of RBCE Metalloproteinase by an Endogenous Inhibitor

A modified SDS-substrate gel method (Herron et al. 1986b) allowed simultaneous visualization of metalloproteinases and their inhibitors in small volumes of unprocessed conditioned medium. SDS-substrate gels were incubated in RSF-conditioned medium that contained active proteinases (see Table 1). Inhibitors present in the electrophoresis sample protect the gelatin substrate from proteinases in the RSF-

Table 2 Secretion of Procollagenase and Prostromelysin by TPA-treated RBCE Cells and RSFs

Time after TPA addition (hr)	Procollagenase (μg protein/10^6 cells)		Prostromelysin (μg protein/10^6 cells)	
	RBCE cells	RSFs	RBCE cells	RSFs
Control[a]	<0.1[b]	<0.1	<0.1	<0.1
24	5.6	15.6	4.1	19.2
48	16.8	30.4	15.2	30.0
56	26.0	n.d.[c]	23.6	n.d.

[a]Control cells were incubated for 48 hr without TPA.
[b]<0.1 μg not detectable by Coomassie blue.
[c]n.d. indicates not determined.

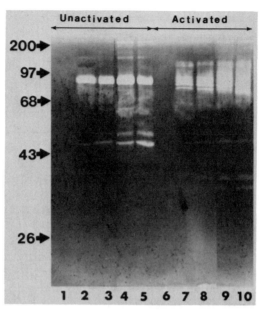

Figure 1 Time course of secretion of metalloproteinase activity by TPA-treated RBCE cells, revealed by SDS-substrate gel analysis. Confluent RBCE cells were cultured in HB101 medium without protein supplement with or without 50 ng/ml TPA, and samples were taken at various times. Aliquots (10 μl) of conditioned medium (CM) were unactivated (lanes *1–5*) or activated with 1 mM APMA for 60 min at 37°C (lanes *6–10*), then electrophoresed on SDS-gelatin gels, incubated, and stained. Areas of clearing represent proteinase activity. (Lanes *1,6*) 56-hr CM from untreated RBCE cells; (lanes *2–5, 7–10*) CM from RBCE cells treated with TPA for 12 hr (lanes *2,7*), 24 hr (lanes *3,8*), 48 hr (lanes *4,9*), or 56 hr (lanes *5,10*). Molecular-weight markers ($M_r \times 10^{-3}$) are shown at the left. (Reprinted, with permission, from Herron et al. 1986b.)

conditioned medium. When conditioned medium from both RBCE cells and RSFs was analyzed, zones showing inhibition of the degradation of the gelatin substrate were observed (Fig. 2). The inhibitory patterns observed in conditioned medium from TPA-treated and untreated RBCE cells and RSFs were quantitatively and qualitatively distinct. Although the major zone of inhibitory activity from both RBCE cells and RSFs migrated at $M_r = 30,000$, two additional inhibitory zones were readily observable in conditioned medium from TPA-treated RBCE cells. The inhibitory zone at $M_r = 19,000$ was seen in conditioned medium from both untreated and TPA-treated RBCE cells and in conditioned medium from TPA-treated RSFs. At this level of detection, the inhibitory zone at $M_r = 22,000$ was seen in conditioned

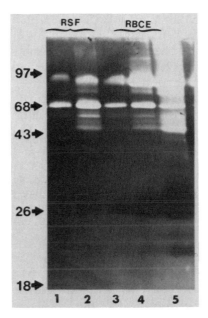

Figure 2 Identification of metalloproteinase inhibitors from RBCE cells and RSFs by SDS-substrate gel analysis. SDS-gelatin gels were used to separate 10-μl aliquots of CM collected from RSFs (lanes *1,2*) or RBCE cells (lanes *3–5*). After removal of SDS, the gels were incubated in medium conditioned by TPA-treated RSFs. Darkened areas represent undigested substrate protected by metalloproteinase inhibitors, and cleared areas represent proteinases resolved during electrophoresis. (Lanes *1,3*) CM from untreated cells; (lane *4*) CM from cells treated with TPA for 24 hr; (lanes *2,5*) CM from cells treated with TPA for 48 hr. Molecular-weight markers ($M_r \times 10^{-3}$) are shown at the left. (Reprinted, with permission, from Herron et al. 1986b.)

medium from untreated and TPA-treated RBCE cells but not in conditioned medium from TPA-treated RSFs.

In control experiments, substrate gels were incubated in a buffer containing the serine proteinase, pancreatic elastase, instead of the metalloproteinase mixture from RSFs. In these gels, no inhibitory zones were found in conditioned medium from RBCE cells, although a zone was present in a lane in which purified human α_1-proteinase inhibitor was separated on the same gel.

The activity of most metalloproteinases is inhibited by a glycoprotein inhibitor (TIMP) ($M_r = 30,000$), which is found in tissue fluids and serum (Murphy et al. 1977, 1983, 1985). To determine whether one of the inhibitory zones in RBCE-conditioned medium could be identified as TIMP, conditioned medium from TPA-stimulated RBCE was treated with antibodies raised against purified rabbit TIMP. The anti-TIMP-affinity resin removed a protein that comigrated with the inhibitory activity at $M_r = 30,000$ on SDS-substrate gels. Indirect evidence thus suggested that the apparent absence of metalloproteinase activities from RBCE-conditioned medium was due to the relatively large concentration of inhibitors present in conditioned medium. To show that TIMP is able to modulate the levels of collagenase and stromelysin activities directly, we incubated unactivated conditioned medium from TPA-treated RBCE cells with anti-TIMP affinity resin and determined metalloproteinase activities after the resin was removed (Table 3). Both collagenase and stromelysin activities were unmasked by the removal of TIMP. Proteinase activity increased after the removal of TIMP, following the same time course as the accumulation of procollagenase and prostromelysin in conditioned medium of RBCE cells (Table 2). Moreover, the actual amount of collagenase and stromelysin activity unmasked by the removal of TIMP was consistent with the concentrations in RSF-conditioned medium (Table 1). Incubation of conditioned medium from TPA-treated RSFs with anti-TIMP-affinity resin had little effect on either enzyme activity, consistent with the low levels of TIMP secreted by these cells (data not shown). These results indicate that the ratio of TIMP to metalloproteinases in RBCE-conditioned medium regulates the expression of proteolytic activity.

Uniform Proteinase and TIMP Expression in a Population of Microvascular Endothelium

Because both metalloproteinases and inhibitors were produced by the same RBCE cultures, it was important to establish whether these proteins were produced by the same cells or by different subpopulations of cells. By indirect immunofluorescence it was clear that virtually all RBCE cells treated with TPA for 24 hours contained intracellular procollagenase (92% of cells), prostromelysin (84% of cells), and TIMP (98% of cells). These data show that RBCE cells are uniformly responsive to TPA and that the expression of connective tissue-degrading proteinase activity is not the property of a subpopulation of RBCE cells. Although RBCE cells were cultured on collagen and secreted matrix components, no immunologically detectable proteinase or TIMP was associated with the extracellular matrix in this experiment.

Table 3 Collagenase and Stromelysin Activities in Conditioned Medium of TPA-treated RBCE Cells before and after Removal of TIMP

Time after TPA addition (hr)	Collagenase (units/10^5 cells)		Stromelysin (units/10^5 cells)	
	TIMP present	TIMP removed	TIMP present	TIMP removed
Control[a]	0	0	0	0
24	0	0	0.8	2.0
48	0	2.5	2.8	7.6
56	0.7	4.2	4.0	11.2

TIMP was removed by incubation of conditioned medium with anti-TIMP-affinity resin.

[a]Control cells were incubated for 56 hr without TPA.

Regulation of Proteinases and Inhibitors in Human Dermal Microvascular Endothelial Cells

We also carried out studies of human dermal microvascular endothelial (HDME) cells to determine whether the regulatory system described above was a peculiarity of rabbit brain microvascular cells. Medium conditioned by variously treated HDME cells and medium conditioned by human dermal fibroblasts were analyzed by SDS-substrate gel electrophoresis and immunoprecipitation of biosynthetically radiolabeled secreted protein with anti-TIMP and anti-collagenase antibodies. These studies showed that HDME cells constitutively secreted high concentrations of TIMP, whereas human dermal fibroblasts did not. Furthermore, TPA-treated HDME cells secreted more than ten times the amount of immunoprecipitable collagenase protein as did untreated HDME cells. Acid-treated human wound fluid and angiogenic fractions isolated from it by TSK-SW4000/3000 gel filtration also stimulated collagenase synthesis and secretion. These fractions did not stimulate the mitogenesis of HDME cells.

Treatment of HDME cells with up to 100 units/ml of purified human interleukin-1 (IL-1) stimulated collagenase synthesis and secretion. However, similar concentrations from the same preparation of IL-1 did not stimulate angiogenesis or HDME cell mitogenesis. This IL-1 did stimulate thymocyte mitogenesis, as expected. These data suggest that although proteinase production may be required for angiogenesis, it is not sufficient.

DISCUSSION

These studies show that microvascular endothelial cells are uniformly capable of synthesizing and secreting the metalloproteinases collagenase and stromelysin, which are likely to be involved in local connective tissue remodeling during the initiation of angiogenesis. The activity of the secreted proteinases was shown to be regulated by the secretion of an endogenous inhibitor of metalloproteinases, TIMP. Rabbit and human microvascular endothelial cells isolated from different capillary beds exhibited similar potential for the secretion of collagenase, stromelysin, and TIMP. Both IL-1, which was not angiogenic, and angiogenic preparations from human wound fluid stimulated proteinase secretion. Therefore, proteinase secretion may be necessary but not sufficient for the initiation of angiogenesis.

ACKNOWLEDGMENTS

This work was supported by grants from the National Institutes of Health (ES07106, AM32746, and GM2734) and by the Office of Health and Environmental Research, United States Department of Energy (DE-AC03-76-SF01012).

REFERENCES

Aggeler, J., S.M. Frisch, and Z. Werb. 1984a. Collagenase is a major gene product of induced rabbit synovial fibroblasts. *J. Cell Biol.* **98:** 1656.

————. 1984b. Changes in cell shape correlate with collagenase gene expression in rabbit synovial fibroblasts. *J. Cell Biol.* **98:** 1662.

Ausprunk, D.H. and J. Folkman. 1977. Migration and proliferation of endothelial cells in preformed and newly formed blood vessels during tumor angiogenesis. *Microvasc. Res.* **14:** 53.

Brinckerhoff, C.E., R.M. McMillan, J.V. Fahey, and E.D. Harris, Jr. 1979. Collagenase production by synovial fibroblasts treated with phorbol myristate acetate. *Arthritis Rheum.* **22:** 1109.

Burger, P.C., D.B. Chandler, and G.K. Klintworth. 1983. Corneal neovascularization as studied by scanning electron microscopy of vascular casts. *Lab. Invest.* **48:** 169.

Chin, J.R., G. Murphy, and Z. Werb. 1985. Stromelysin, a connective tissue-degrading metalloendopeptidase secreted by stimulated rabbit synovial fibroblasts in parallel with collagenase. Biosynthesis, isolation, characterization, and substrates. *J. Biol. Chem.* **260:** 12367.

Folkman, J. 1984. What is the role of endothelial cells in angiogenesis? *Lab. Invest.* **51:** 601.

Galloway, W.A., G. Murphy, J.D. Sandy, J. Gavrilovic, T.E. Cawston, and J.J. Reynolds. 1983. Purification and characterization of a rabbit bone metalloproteinase that degrades proteoglycan and other connective-tissue components. *Biochem. J.* **209:** 741.

Gross, J.L., D. Moscatelli, and D.B. Rifkin. 1983. Increased capillary endothelial cell protease activity in response to angiogenic stimuli *in vitro*. *Proc. Natl. Acad. Sci.* **80:** 2623.

Gross, J., J.H. Highberger, B. Johnson-Wint, and C. Biswas. 1980. Mode of action and regulation of tissue collagenases. In *Collagenase in normal and pathological connective tissues* (ed. D.E. Woolley and J.M. Evanson), p. 11. John Wiley, Chichester.

Gross, J.L., D. Moscatelli, E.A. Jaffe, and D.B. Rifkin. 1982. Plasminogen activator and collagenase production by cultured capillary endothelial cells. *J. Cell Biol.* **95:** 974.

Herron, G.S., Z. Werb, K. Dwyer, and M.J. Banda. 1986a. Secretion of metalloproteinases by stimulated capillary endothelial cells. I. Production of procollagenase and prostromelysin exceeds expression of proteolytic activity. *J. Biol. Chem.* **261:** 2810.

Herron, G.S., M.J. Banda, E.J. Clark, J. Gavrilovic, and Z. Werb. 1986b. Secretion of metalloproteinases by capillary endothelial cells. II. Expression of collagenase and stromelysin activities is regulated by endogenous inhibitors. *J. Biol. Chem.* **261:** 2814.

Kalebic, T., S. Garbisa, B. Glaser, and L.A. Liotta. 1983. Basement membrane collagen: Degradation by migrating endothelial cells. *Science* **221:** 281.

Kramer, R.H., G.-M. Fuh, and M.A. Karasek. 1985. Type IV collagen synthesis by cultured human microvascular endothelial cells and its deposition into the subendothelial basement membrane. *Biochemistry* **24:** 7423.

Madri, J.A. and S.K. Williams. 1983. Capillary endothelial cell cultures: Phenotypic modulation by matrix components. *J. Cell Biol.* **97**: 153.

Moscatelli, D.A., D.B. Rifkin, and E.A. Jaffe. 1985. Production of latent collagenase by human umbilical vein endothelial cells in response to angiogenic preparations. *Exp. Cell Res.* **156**: 379.

Murphy, G. and J.J. Reynolds. 1985. Current views of collagen degradation. Progress towards understanding the resorption of connective tissues. *BioEssays* **2**: 55.

Murphy, G., E.C. Cartwright, A. Sellers, and J.J. Reynolds. 1977. The detection and characterisation of collagenase inhibitors from rabbit tissues in culture. *Biochim. Biophys. Acta* **483**: 493.

Murphy, G., T.E. Cawston, W.A. Galloway, M.J. Barnes, R.A.D. Bunning, E. Mercer, J.J. Reynolds, and R.E. Burgeson. 1983. Metalloproteinases from rabbit bone culture medium degrades types IV and V collagens, laminin and fibronectin. *Biochem. J.* **199**: 807.

Sage, H., P. Pritzl, and P. Bornstein. 1981. Secretory phenotypes of endothelial cells in culture: Comparison of aortic, venous, capillary, and corneal endothelium. *Arteriosclerosis* **1**: 427.

Sellers, A., E. Cartwright, G. Murphy, and J.J. Reynolds. 1977. Evidence that latent collagenases are enzyme-inhibitor complexes. *Biochem. J.* **163**: 303.

Stricklin, G.P., E.A. Bauer, J.J. Jeffrey, and A.Z. Eisen. 1977. Human skin collagenase: Isolation of precursor and active forms from both fibroblast and organ cultures. *Biochemistry* **16**: 1607.

Studies on the Regulation of Protease Activity during Cell Invasion and Angiogenesis

D.B. Rifkin, O. Saksela, D. Moscatelli,
M. Presta,* P. Mignatti,[†] and L. Ossowski[‡]

Department of Cell Biology, New York University Medical Center
New York, New York 10016

[‡]Department of Cellular Physiology and Immunology
The Rockefeller University, New York, New York 10021

We have recently described the isolation from term placenta of a human form of basic fibroblast growth factor (bFGF) that is angiogenic in vivo and induces the production of the proteases plasminogen activator (PA) and collagenase in bovine capillary endothelial cells (BCE) (Moscatelli et al. 1986). The structure and molecular biology of this molecule are described by Sommer et al. (this volume), and certain biological properties of the protein and its receptor are described by Moscatelli et al. (this volume). We have focused on the regulation of proteases secreted by endothelial cells because one of the early processes in angiogenesis is the dissolution of the capillary basement membrane and the subsequent movement of endothelial cells through this breach in the basement membrane (Ausprunk and Folkman 1977). We have found that the increased production of proteases by endothelial cells exposed to bFGF may be controlled at both the level of synthesis and the level of activity.

Effect of Transforming Growth Factor-β

In fibroblasts, the production of PA can be blocked by transforming growth factor-β (TGF-β), which has also been shown to be potent inhibitor of epithelial cell proliferation (Keski-Oja et al. 1986). Picogram quantities of TGF-β added to cultures of BCE simultaneously with bFGF suppress the normally observed increase in PA activity. The effect is both dose- and time-dependent; the effective dose of TGF-β required to neutralize PA stimulation after bFGF exposure increases as the time between bFGF and TGF-β exposure increases. The stimula-

Present addresses: *Institute of General Pathology, University of Brescia, Via Valsabbina 19, 25124 Brescia, Italy; [†]Department of Genetics and Microbiology, University of Pavia, Via S. Epifanio 14, 27100 Pavia, Italy.

tory effect of bFGF cannot be completely abolished by increasing the amount of TGF-β, but the inhibition by TFG-β is greatly enhanced when the cells are pretreated for 1–3 hours with TGF-β before addition of bFGF. If the preincubation time with TGF-β is 6 hours, the inhibition of the bFGF effect on PA levels is almost complete. Sequential changes of serum-containing medium during a 6-hour period prior to exposure to bFGF blocks the effect of bFGF. Conversely, bFGF is able to stimulate PA production in cells exposed to TGF-β and which consequently have PA levels below the basal level normally found in BCE. The inhibitory effect of TGF-β is transient, and the cells recover basal levels of PA production about 16 hours after exposure to TGF-β. The effect of bFGF lasts longer and PA production is increased fivefold to tenfold above normal for at least 3 days after exposure to bFGF.

TGF-β exerts its inhibitory effect on PA levels by two mechanisms. First, there is a decrease in PA synthesis, as shown by fibrinolysis assays and zymography. Second, there is an increase in the synthesis of a PA inhibitor, as shown by reverse zymography and by immunoprecipitation with an antiserum to an inhibitor of PA. TGF-β does not alter the binding of radiolabeled bFGF to its receptor. Thus, bFGF and TGF-β may act together to modulate PA production by endothelial cells. Since platelets contain the highest levels of TGF-β of any cell types, TGF-β released during clot formation or wound healing may suppress the basal PA production of endothelial cells and ensure the initial formation of a clot. After 24 hours, the TGF-β is no longer effective and PA production will recover. If bFGF is liberated by endothelial cells or other cells in the area of a thrombus or wound, this would promote subsequent fibrin lysis, mitosis, and cell movement.

Protease Inhibitors and Cellular Invasion
A second mechanism for controlling proteolytic activity is via extracellular inhibitors of proteolysis. The avascularity of cartilage is proposed to result from high levels of protease inhibitors within the cartilagenous matrix, which would prevent endothelial cells from penetrating into the tissue (Langer et al. 1980). To understand the role of proteases and protease inhibitors in the regulation of cell invasion, we have conducted a series of experiments to monitor the effect of specific protease inhibitors on cell invasion through the human amnion membrane. Fresh human amnion membrane was stretched over Teflon rings and then held in place with a silicon O-ring, thus forming a chamber within the Teflon ring, with the epithelial side of the amnion as the bottom of the chamber. The epithelium was removed and the chambers were placed on supports in 35-mm petri dishes. The effects on cell invasion of inhibitors of metallo-, serine- and cysteine-proteases added to the

111

culture medium were monitored using [^{125}I]iododeoxyuridine-labeled cells placed on the amnion. Initial experiments were performed using the highly invasive clone B16/BL6 of the B16 melanoma line.

Invasion was quantitated by measuring the radioactivity associated with the amniotic membrane after the cells remaining on the surface of the basement membrane were removed by lysis and scraping. The results obtained with protease inhibitors as well as specific antisera showed that inhibition of collagenase and plasmin prevented invasion of the amnion (Mignatti et al. 1986). A low-molecular-weight inhibitor of collagenase is able to block invasion even when added to the stromal side of the amnion. Tissue invasion is also blocked by antibodies to urokinase. On the contrary, antibodies to tissue PA, as well as inhibitors of cysteine proteases, are ineffective in blocking invasion.

These results suggest that urokinase activates plasminogen to plasmin and that plasmin converts procollagenase to collagenase. This hypothesis predicts that collagenase produced in the absence of plasmin and/or urokinase should promote invasion of the amnion. Indeed, Mersalyl, a compound known to activate collagenase, stimulates invasion under conditions where plasmin formation and/or activity are blocked. Endothelial cells stimulated by bFGF also invade the amniotic membrane, although the number of cells that invade is much lower than that observed with the B16/Bl6 cells.

Preliminary experiments with the collagenase inhibitor in combination with bFGF on the chick chorioallantoic membrane indicate that collagenase activity may be a prerequisite for invasion during angiogenesis as well as during tumor cell invasion.

CONCLUSIONS

These results indicate that the positive effect of bFGF on the invasive potential of endothelial cells may be modulated in at least two ways. Molecules such as TGF-β may suppress the synthesis of the proteases required for tissue lysis, whereas high local levels of protease inhibitors may block the activity of those enzymes produced by the stimulated cells. Therefore, the observed reponse to an angiogenesis factor must be the net effect of both positive and negative controlling molecules.

ACKNOWLEDGMENTS

This work was supported by grants from the National Institutes of Health, American Cancer Society, Juvenile Diabetes Society, and the Council for Tobacco Research, Inc.

REFERENCES
Ausprunk, D. and J. Folkman. 1977. Migration and proliferation of endotheli-

al cells in preformed and newly formed blood vessels during tumor angio-genesis. *Microvasc. Res.* **14**: 53.

Keski-Oja, J., E.B. Loef, R.M. Lyons, R.J. Coffey, and H.L. Moses. 1986. The transforming growth factors and control of neoplastic cell growth. *J. Cell. Biochem.* (in press).

Langer, R., H. Conn, J. Vacanti, C. Haudenschild, and J. Folkman. 1980. Control of tumor growth in animals by infusion of an angiogenesis inhibitor. *Proc. Natl. Acad. Sci.* **77**: 4331.

Mignatti, P., E. Robbins, and D.B. Rifkin. 1986. Tumor invasion through the human amniotic membrane: Requirement for a proteinase cascade. *Cell* **47**: 487.

Moscatelli, D., M. Presta, and D.B. Rifkin. 1986. Purification of a factor from human placenta that stimulates capillary endothelial cell protease produc-tion, DNA synthesis, and migration. *Proc. Natl. Acad. Sci.* **83**: 2091.

113

Retinal Pigment Epithelial Cells Release Inhibitors of Neovascularization

B.M. Glaser, P.A. Campochiaro,* J.L. Davis, Jr., and J. Jerdan

Center for Vitreoretinal Research, Wilmer Ophthalmological Institute
Johns Hopkins University, Baltimore, Maryland 21205

*University of Virginia, Department of Ophthalmology
Charlottesville, Virginia 22903

Neovascularization plays a crucial role in the pathogenesis of several important human disorders, including diabetic retinopathy, retinopathy of prematurity, choroidal neovascularization (age-related macular degeneration, histoplasmosis, etc.), sickle cell retinopathy, tumor growth, and rheumatoid arthritis. The possibility that controlling neovascularization will aid in the treatment of these disorders has prompted an extensive search for inhibitors of new blood vessel formation (Folkman 1971). Most inhibitors of neovascularization so far identified have been extracted from tissues that are avascular, i.e., cartilage (Eisenstein et al. 1973; Brem and Folkman 1975; Sorgente et al. 1975; Langer et al. 1976), vitreous (Brem et al. 1977; Lutty et al. 1983), and lens (Williams et al. 1984). Unfortunately, the study of these inhibitors is severely limited by the fact that only small quantities of active material can be extracted from these sources (Lee and Langer 1983).

It has been suggested that diabetic intraocular neovascularization is less likely to occur in eyes with chorioretinal scars (Beetham et al. 1969). This has led to the widespread use of argon laser and xenon photocoagulation to therapeutically induce chorioretinal scar formation. The production of these scars often results in the rapid regression of intraocular neovascularization in eyes with proliferative diabetic retinopathy (Beetham et al. 1969; Doft and Blankenship 1984). Regression occurs even when photocoagulation and resultant chorioretinal scarring are located in areas remote from the new blood vessels (Beetham et al. 1969; Diabetic Retinopathy Study Group 1978; Foulds 1980; Weiter and Zuckerman 1980; Stefansson et al. 1983; Doft and Blankenship 1984). Retinal pigment epithelial (RPE) cells are one component of these scars. We have shown that human RPE cells in culture release a substance (or substances) that causes the regression of new blood vessels on the chick embryonic yolk sac and inhibits vascular endothelial cell proliferation in vitro (Glaser et al. 1985).

DISCUSSION

Chorioretinal scars are mainly composed of astrocytes, RPE cells, and possibly fibroblasts (Wallow and Tsa 1973; Wallow et al. 1973; Wallow and Davis 1979). In our experiments, human RPE cells in culture, but not astrocytes or corneal fibroblasts, released a substance (or substances) that caused the regression of new blood vessels on the chick embryonic yolk sac. Vessels appear in the chick embryonic yolk sac at 48 hours and grow rapidly over the next 6–8 days (Taylor and Folkman 1982). Therefore, the vasculature of the 4–5-day-old embryos used in our studies was in an actively developing or "neovascular" mode. Inhibitors of neovascularization derived from cartilage (Eisenstein et al. 1975), aorta (Goren et al. 1977), and lens (Williams et al. 1984) also inhibit proliferation of vascular endothelial cells. We have found that RPE-conditioned media, but not astrocyte- or fibroblast-conditioned media, inhibited the proliferation of fetal bovine aortic endothelial cells and human retinal microvessel endothelial cells. The effect of RPE-conditioned media on the proliferation of endothelial cells was reversible and was not associated with cell death. In contrast, RPE-conditioned media enhanced the proliferation of fibroblasts in culture.

The inability of astrocytes and fibroblasts to release detectable levels of substances that cause the regression of new blood vessels and inhibit the proliferation of vascular endothelial cells demonstrates the relative uniqueness of human RPE cells in this regard. However, it does not indicate that other cell types, cells from other species, or cells under other conditions might not release similar substances. These possibilities are currently being addressed in our laboratory.

Cell-cell interactions play an important role in a large number of biologic processes, including those that occur during development, wound healing, and tumor growth and spread. The establishment and control of an adequate blood supply has a role in all of these processes. Therefore, cell-cell interactions are also likely to be involved in controlling new blood vessel formation and regression during these processes. The ability of RPE cells to inhibit the proliferation of vascular endothelial cells and to induce the regression of new blood vessels may be important during ocular development, since the RPE cells lie between the extremely vascular choroid and the avascular outer retina. RPE cells in a laser-induced chorioretinal scar may release the same substance into the vitreous cavity to cause regression of intraocular new blood vessels. Previous studies (Glaser et al. 1980) have shown that retina, under certain conditions, can release a stimulator of neovascularization. It is therefore of significant interest that RPE cells, although derived from the same neuroectoderm as the remainder of the retina, release inhibitors of neovascularization.

The release of the inhibitor of vascular endothelial cell proliferation is dependent upon RPE cell density. RPE cells in confluent cultures release less inhibitor than RPE cells in subconfluent cultures. Several days after RPE cells reach confluence, the release of inhibitor once again increases. Corresponding to the increase in inhibitor release, RPE cells begin to overgrow the monolayer to form localized regions with multiple cell layers. The effect of cell density on inhibitor release possibly depends upon the cell-cell relationships and associated cellular morphology. RPE cells in subconfluent and superconfluent cultures do not maintain the highly ordered cell-cell relationships present within the RPE monolayer in the normal eye. Alterations in the highly ordered RPE monolayer that occur in chorioretinal scars and that are possibly mimicked in superconfluent and subconfluent RPE cultures may result in the enhancement of inhibitor release. This may occur despite the fact that some RPE cells are destroyed by the photocoagulation, since it is the remaining cells that can then undergo alterations in morphology. The resultant enhancement in the release of inhibitor into the adjacent retina and vitreous may play a role in the effect of photocoagulation-induced chorioretinal scarring on the regression and prevention of neovascularization in diabetic retinopathy. Further studies of the relationship between inhibitor release and RPE cell morphology and environment are under way in our laboratory.

Other inhibitors of neovascularization so far studied have their effect on actively proliferating vessels but do not cause regression of established vessels (Taylor and Folkman 1982). Therefore, inhibitors potentially released by normal RPE cells would not be expected to cause regression of the nonproliferating, established capillary bed of the choroid. However, small amounts of RPE-cell-derived inhibitor may prevent any inadvertent new blood vessel formation from the choriocapillaries. In senile macular degeneration, one might speculate that the RPE cells may suffer a biochemical defect, even in the absence of morphologic alterations, so that the level of inhibitor production is reduced and new blood vessel invasion from the choriocapillaries becomes more likely.

SUMMARY

We have described, for the first time, a pigment epithelial-cell-derived substance (or substances) that stimulates the regression of new blood vessels on the chick embryonic yolk sac and inhibits FBAE and human retinal microvessel endothelial cell proliferation. This discovery raises several interesting possibilities that require further investigation. Under normal conditions, RPE cells and Bruch's membrane are positioned as a barrier between the highly vascular choriocapillaries and the avascular outer retina. The ability of RPE cells to release an inhibitor of vascular endothelial cell proliferation may provide the biochemical mechanism by which the barrier functions. Since cell-cell relationships seem to alter inhibitor release by RPE cells, photocoagulation and subsequent chorioretinal scarring may function by altering the local architecture and morphology of the RPE cells so that increased levels of the inhibitor may be achieved in the surrounding retina and vitreous, thereby inhibiting vessel formation in proliferative diabetic retinopathy. Most importantly, further study of the interaction between RPE cells and the vasculature is likely to be fruitful in improving our understanding of neovascularization and suggesting new approaches to its management.

REFERENCES

Beetham, W.P., L.M. Aiello, and M.C. Balodimos. 1969. Ruby-laser photocoagulation of early diabetic neovascular retinopathy: Preliminary report of a long-term controlled study. *Trans. Am. Ophthalmol. Soc.* **67**: 39.

Brem, H. and J. Folkman. 1975. Inhibition of tumor angiogenesis mediated by cartilage. *J. Exp. Med.* **141**: 427.

Brem, S., I. Preis, and R. Langer. 1977. Inhibition of neovascularization by an extract derived from vitreous. *Am. J. Ophthalmol.* **84**: 323.

Diabetic Retinopathy Study Group. 1978. Photocoagulation treatment of proliferative diabetic retinopathy: The second report of diabetic retinopathy findings. *Ophthalmology* **85**: 82.

Doft, B.H. and G. Blankenship. 1984. Retinopathy risk factor regression after laser panretinal photocoagulation for proliferative diabetic retinopathy. *Ophthalmology* **91**: 1453.

Eisenstein, R., K.E. Kuettner, and C. Neopolitan. 1975. The resistance of certain tissues to invasion. III. Cartilage extracts inhibit the growth of fibroblasts and endothelial cells in culture. *Am. J. Pathol.* **81**: 337.

Eisenstein, R., N. Sorgente, and L.W. Soble. 1973. The resistance of certain tissues to invasion. Penetrability of explanted tissues by vascular mesenchyme. *Am. J. Pathol.* **73**: 765.

Folkman, J. 1971. Tumor angiogenesis: Therapeutic implications. *N. Engl. J. Med.* **285**: 1182.

Foulds, W.S. 1980. The role of photocoagulation in the treatment of retinal disease. *Trans. Ophthalmol. Soc. N. Z.* **32**: 82.

Glaser, B.M., P.A. D'Amore, and R.G. Michels. 1980. Demonstration of vasoproliferative activity from mammalian retina. *J. Cell Biol.* **840**: 298.

Glaser, B.M., P.A. Campochiaro, J.L. Davis, and M. Sato. 1985. Retinal pigment epithelial cells release an inhibitor of neovascularization. *Arch. Ophthalmol.* **103**: 1870.

Goren, S.B., R. Eisenstein, and E. Chromokos. 1977. The inhibition of corneal vascularization in rabbits. *Am. J. Ophthalmol.* **84**: 305.

Langer, R., H. Brem, and K. Falterman. 1976. Isolation of a cartilage factor that inhibits tumor neovascularization. *Science* **19**: 70.

Lee, A. and R. Langer. 1983. Shark cartilage contains inhibitors of tumor angiogenesis. *Science* **221**: 1185.

Lutty, G.A., D.C. Thompson, and J.Y. Gallup. 1983. Vitreous: An inhibitor of retinal-extract induced neovascularization. *Invest. Ophthalmol.* **24**: 52.

Sorgente, N., K.E. Kuettner, and L.W. Soble. 1975. The resistance of certain tissues to invasion. II. Evidence for extractable factors in cartilage which inhibit invasion by vascularized mesenchyme. *Lab. Invest.* **32**: 217.

Stefansson, E., M.B. Landers, and M.L. Wolbarsht. 1983. Oxygenation and vasodilation in relation to diabetic and other proliferative retinopathies. *Ophthalmic Surg.* **14**: 209.

Taylor, S. and J. Folkman. 1982. Protamine is an inhibitor of angiogenesis. *Nature* **297**: 307.

Wallow, I.H.L. and M.D. Davis. 1979. Clinicopathologic correlation of xenon arc and argon laser photocoagulation procedure in human diabetic eyes. *Arch. Ophthalmol.* **97**: 2308.

Wallow, I.H.L. and M.O.M. Tso. 1973. Repair after xenon arc photocoagulation 3. An electron microscopic study of the evolution of retinal lesions in rhesus monkeys. *Am. J. Ophthalmol.* **75**: 957.

Wallow, I.H.L., M.O.M. Tso, and B.S. Fine. 1973. Retinal repair after experimental xenon arc photocoagulation. I. A comparison between rhesus monkey and rabbit. *Am. J. Ophthalmol.* **75**: 32.

Weiter, J.J. and R. Zuckerman. 1980. The influence of the photoreceptor-RPE complex on the inner retina. An explanation for the beneficial effects of photocoagulation. *Ophthalmology* **87**: 1133.

Williams, G.A., R. Eisenstein, and B. Schumacher. 1984. Inhibitor of vascular endothelial cell growth in the lens. *Am. J. Ophthalmol.* **97**: 366.

Inhibitors of Endothelial Cell Proliferation

P. Böhlen, M. Fràter-Schroeder, T. Michel, and Z.-P. Jiang

Biochemisches Institut, Universität Zürich
CH-8057 Zürich, Switzerland

Angiogenesis or neovascularization is a complex physiological process that primarily involves migration, proliferation, and differentiation of endothelial cells. It occurs normally during mammalian development (embryogenesis and organ growth) and cyclically in adult females (e.g., development of the corpus luteum), but hardly in adult males. On the other hand, angiogenesis readily occurs in adults during wound healing and in a large variety of pathophysiological conditions. This suggests that angiogenesis is a tightly controlled physiological event. Little is known about the molecular mechanisms involved in the regulation of angiogenesis. Soluble factors that either stimulate or inhibit individual events necessary for the process of angiogenesis, such as the migration or proliferation of endothelial cells, could participate in those regulatory pathways. The existence of stimulatory factors in many tissues has long been known, and more recently, several proteins with mitogenic and/or angiogenic activity (basic and acidic fibroblast growth factors, transforming growth factor-α, angiogenin) have been purified to homogeneity and structurally characterized. Likewise, many tissues contain inhibitors of endothelial cell proliferation or angiogenesis (for references, see Fràter-Schroeder et al. 1986), but none of those inhibitory activities have been structurally defined so far. In an attempt to characterize molecules that are potentially inhibitory regulators of angiogenesis, we have employed an in vitro growth assay using cultured bovine aortic endothelial cells (BAECs) to identify novel natural inhibitors of endothelial cell proliferation. We present here our results on the characterization of several endothelial cell growth inhibitors. Since inhibitory activity on endothelial cells in vitro does not necessarily correlate with inhibition of angiogenesis in vivo, we have also begun to investigate the effects of those defined growth inhibitors on neovascularization.

RESULTS
Transforming Growth Factor-β
Although transforming growth factor-β (TGF-β) was initially thought

to be a mitogenic protein because it can induce anchorage-independent and monolayer growth in certain cells, more recent data indicate that TGF-β can also act as a potent inhibitor of cell growth. We have shown that TGF-β isolated from human or porcine platelets inhibits the proliferation of BAECs in vitro (Fràter-Schroeder et al. 1986). Half-maximal inhibition of basal endothelial cell growth (proliferation in DMEM/10% calf serum, in the absence of exogenously added growth factor) occurred over a dose range of 0.01–3 ng/ml, with a half-maximally active dose of about 0.5 ng/ml. Growth stimulated with basic fibroblast growth factor (bFGF; 0.9 ng/ml, a nearly maximally stimulating dose) was antagonized by TGF-β at identical doses. This antagonism appears to be of a noncompetitive nature, since it could not be counteracted by even very high doses of bFGF (10 ng/ml), and the dose of TGF-β needed for half-maximal growth inhibition remained constant regardless of bFGF concentration. TGF-β-induced inhibition of endothelial cell proliferation is reversible: Nonconfluent cells exposed to TGF-β for 5 days, after removal of the inhibitor, resumed growth at a rate indistinguishable from that of control cells. Low cytotoxicity of TGF-β for endothelial cells was also suggested by the absence of cell shedding when confluent cells were exposed to the inhibitor for periods of up to 16 days. Such long-term exposure only affected the morphology of the cells, as evidenced by the disappearance of the typical cobblestone pattern of confluent endothelial cell layers (upon removal of inhibitor the normal cobblestone morphology was reestablished).

Interferons

Recombinant bovine interferon-α1 (IFN-α1), IFN-β2, and IFN-γ were found to be inhibitory for cultured BAECs (Fig. 1). Proliferation was inhibited in a dose-dependent manner regardless of whether basal growth with serum alone or bFGF-stimulated growth was investigated. Among the interferons, IFN-γ was highly potent, whereas the other interferons were considerably less active. Interestingly, the inhibitory potencies of IFNs were higher for bFGF-stimulated cells than for cells proliferating in the presence of serum alone. Furthermore, IFN-α and IFN-β had a small but consistent stimulatory activity upon endothelial cells growing in serum/medium alone (130% of control). The action of IFNs was not cytotoxic, as determined by an indium-release assay using high IFN doses (125 ng/ml IFN-γ).

Tumor Necrosis Factor

Human recombinant tumor necrosis factor-α (TNF-α) also inhibited the proliferation of BAECs. Basal cell growth and FGF-stimulated cell

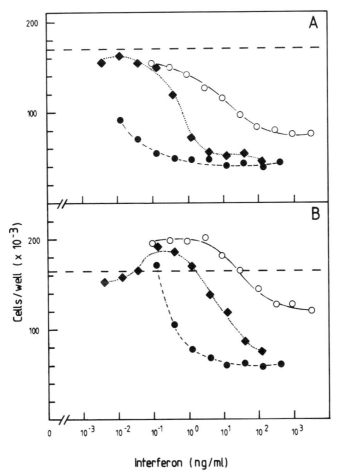

Figure 1 Inhibition of endothelial cell proliferation by interferons. (*A*) bFGF-stimulated cell proliferation (0.9 ng/ml bFGF); (*B*) basal cell proliferation. (○) IFN-α1; (●) IFN-γ; (■) IFN-β2. Dashed line indicates growth of control cells.

growth were inhibited with TNF doses ranging from 0.1 to 10 ng/ml (half-maximally inhibitory concentration: 0.5–1 ng/ml). The mitogenic activities of basic and acidic FGFs were antagonized equally by TNF. The antimitogenic effect of TNF was not specific for BAECs, as the proliferation of bovine brain capillary endothelial cells and bovine smooth-muscle cells was also inhibited. As with TGF-β, the inhibitory effect of TNF could not be overcome by high doses of bFGF, indicating that this antagonism is of a noncompetitive nature. The TNF effect on endothelial cells was reversible when the inhibitor was removed from the culture medium. TNF, at supramaximal concentration of 140 ng/ml, did not induce the release of radioactive indium from prelabeled cells, nor did it cause shedding of cells from confluent monolayers in long-term (10-day) culture. This suggests that the inhibitory activity of TNF is not caused by cytotoxicity.

In collaboration with W. Risau and R. Hallmann (Tübingen), the activity of TNF on angiogenesis in vivo was tested in the rabbit cornea assay. In contrast to its inhibitory activity on endothelial cells in vitro, TNF did not inhibit bFGF-stimulated angiogenesis in vivo. On the contrary, TNF (1 μg implanted in the cornea in a polymer pellet) had noticeable angiogenic properties. Furthermore, TNF potentiated in a dose-dependent manner bFGF-induced angiogenesis (0.3 μg bFGF, 1 or 10 μg TNF). TNF also produced an inflammatory response at the site of implantation.

DISCUSSION

TGF-β, IFNs, and TNF are well-known regulatory proteins whose physiological significance was originally thought to be associated with first-recognized biological activities, i.e., transforming, antiviral, and necrotic/cytotoxic activities, respectively. Although it is now well established (Hunter 1986) that those factors are also antimitogenic for a variety of cell types in culture (mostly transformed cells, but also some normal cells), it remains unclear whether this activity bears physiological significance in the control of cell growth. In this context, the observation that TGF-β, IFNs, and TNF are potent inhibitors of endothelial cell proliferation in vitro is of interest. The growth-inhibitory activity of TGF-β has recently been studied in some detail (Baird and Durkin 1986; Fràter-Schroeder et al. 1986; Heimark et al. 1986). The endothelial cell inhibitory activities of IFN-α and TNF have also been reported (Heyns et al. 1985; Sato et al. 1986; Stolpen et al. 1986), but so far the antimitogenic activities of IFNs and TNF have not been studied in sufficient detail. Our in vitro data on those types of inhibitors extend the previously existing information.

The finding that the potent inhibitor of endothelial cell growth in vitro, TNF, does not apparently have a similar effect in vivo is noteworthy. Although inhibitory activities on endothelial cell proliferation in vitro and in vivo (neovascularization) do not need to correlate, it is somewhat surprising to find a clear stimulatory/potentiating effect of TNF on angiogenesis. It is conceivable that this angiogenic response of TNF is caused indirectly by the inflammatory reaction. However, more work is required to clarify the mechanisms involved.

A number of questions need to be addressed in future research. First, what are the mechanisms of action with respect to the antimitogenic effects of TGF-β, IFNs, and TNF on endothelial cells? Apart from the apparently noncompetitive nature of the interaction between inhibitors and bFGF, nothing is known as to how those potent inhibitors act. It will be of interest to establish, for example, whether cross-modulation of receptors for growth signals is involved or whether at least some of the inhibitors act through induction of IFN-β mRNA and protein, as has recently been shown to be the case with respect to the action of TNF on fibroblasts (Kohase et al. 1986). Furthermore, it will be important to determine whether any of various uncharacterized endothelial cell growth or angiogenesis inhibitors (see above) are identical to either TGF-β, IFNs, or TNF. At least TGF-β is a rather ubiquitously occurring protein, and it is therefore conceivable that some of the inhibitory activities described may correspond to this factor. It is also quite clear that additional inhibitory substances can be found in tissues. For example, at least two additional inhibitors not apparently related to known factors may exist in platelets in addition to TGF-β (Brown and Clemmons 1986; D. Huber and P. Böhlen, unpubl.). Moreover, it should be mentioned that other known substances, e.g., protamine, heparin, and heparin derivatives are inhibitors of endothelial cell growth and/or angiogenesis and deserve to be studied further, both in vitro and in vivo. Finally, we need to study the physiological significance of the currently known inhibitors. In this context, a better understanding is necessary of the extent to which there is a correlation between the in vivo and in vitro actions of potential inhibitors. This should help to clarify whether inhibitors identified by in vitro methods are reasonable candidates for inhibitors of angiogenesis.

ACKNOWLEDGMENTS

We thank Drs. W. Risau and R. Hallmann (Max-Planck-Institut for Developmental Biology, Tübingen, Federal Republic of Germany) for carrying out angiogenesis assays. We also thank Drs. F. Frickel (Knoll GmbH, Ludwigshafen, Federal Republic of Germany) and R. Steiger (CIBA-GEIGY, Basel, Switzerland) for gifts of human recombinant TNF and bovine recombinant interferons, respectively. Drs. D. Gospodarowicz and W. Risau kindly provided bovine capillary endothelial cells and smooth-muscle cells, respectively. Research was supported by the Kanton of Zürich, the Swiss National Science Foundation (grant 3.649-0.84), the EMDO Foundation, Zürich, and the Jubiläums-Stiftung of the University of Zürich.

REFERENCES
Baird, A. and T. Durkin. 1986. Inhibition of endothelial cell proliferation by type-beta transforming growth factor. *Biochem. Biophys. Res. Commun.* **138:** 476.

Brown, M. and D. Clemmons. 1986. Platelets contain a peptide inhibitor of endothelial cell replication and growth. *Proc. Natl. Acad. Sci.* **83**: 3321.

Fràter-Schroeder, M., G. Müller, W. Birchmeier, and P. Böhlen. 1986. Transforming growth factor-beta inhibits endothelial cell proliferation. *Biochem. Biophys. Res. Commun.* **137**: 295.

Heimark, R., D. Twardzik, and S. Schwartz. 1986. Inhibition of endothelial regeneration by type-beta transforming growth factor from platelets. *Science* **233**: 1078.

Heyns, A., A. Eldor, I. Vlodavsky, N. Kaiser, R. Fridman, and A. Panet. 1985. The antiproliferative effect of interferon and the mitogenic activity of growth factors are independent cell cycle events. Studies with vascular smooth muscle cells and endothelial cells. *Exp. Cell Res.* **161**: 297.

Hunter, T. 1986. Cell growth control mechanisms. *Nature* **322**: 14.

Kohase, M., D. Henriksen-DeStefano, L. Tay, J. Vilcek, and P. Sehgal. 1986. Induction of beta2-interferon by tumor necrosis factor: A homeostatic mechanism in the control of cell proliferation. *Cell* **45**: 659.

Sato, N., T. Goto, K. Haranaka, N. Satomi, H. Nariuchi, Y. Mano-Hirano, and Y. Sawasaki. 1986. Actions of tumor necrosis factor on cultured vascular endothelial cells: Morphologic modulation, growth inhibition, and cytotoxicity. *J. Natl. Cancer Inst.* **76**: 1113.

Stolpen, A., E. Guinan, W. Fiers, and J. Pober. 1986. Recombinant tumor necrosis factor and immune interferon act singly and in combination to reorganize human vascular endothelial cell monolayers. *Am. J. Pathol.* **123**: 16.

124

The Role of the Pericyte in Microvascular Growth Control

P.A. D'Amore and A. Orlidge

The Children's Hospital and Harvard Medical School
Boston, Massachusetts 02115

The growth of the microvasculature is remarkably well controlled, with turnover rates of 90 days to 30 years reported for the endothelial cells (ECs) of various microvascular beds (Hobson and Denekamp 1984). The regulators that are responsible for this stringent growth control are not known. However, studies of control mechanisms in other cell systems implicate growth factors, extracellular matrix, and cell-cell interactions.

With respect to the cell-cell interactions, a number of clinical and experimental observations suggest that the pericyte may act in vivo to suppress capillary EC growth. We have established cultures of microvascular ECs and pericytes and have used these cells to examine the possibility that pericytes can modulate the proliferation of capillary ECs.

Isolation and Identification of Microvascular Cells

Microvascular ECs and pericytes were isolated from retina and adrenal gland using modifications (Gitlin and D'Amore 1983) of the methods described by Folkman et al. (1979). The techniques involved controlled enzyme digestion of minced tissues to release the capillary fragments. The isolated fragments were then cultured on gelatin-coated tissue culture plastic in the presence of heparin-binding growth factors to select for EC growth or on uncoated plastic in medium supplemented with fetal calf serum (FCS) to select for pericyte growth. The identity of the ECs was established by demonstrating the ability of the cells to take up acetylated low-density lipoprotein (LDL) and to stain with antisera to von Willebrand's factor (VWF). Pericytes were differentiated from ECs by their inability to take up acetylated LDL and by the absence of staining with VWF antisera. They were further distinguished from smooth-muscle cells (SMCs) by the lack of "hill-and-valley" growth pattern at confluence and by their expression of both muscle and non-muscle actin isotypes (in contrast to SMCs, which contain predominantly muscle actins) (Herman and D'Amore 1985).

125

Coculture of ECs and Pericytes with Direct Contact

Capillary ECs and pericytes were cocultured in a system that allowed contact between the cells. The pericytes were growth-arrested by mitomycin treatment prior to coculture, so that any change in cell number that occurred in these cocultures could be attributed to ECs. In the first series of experiments, pericytes and ECs (at a ratio of 1 : 1) were cocultured for 2 weeks. At each time point, the cells of quadruplicate wells containing mitomycin-treated pericytes alone, ECs alone, or ECs cocultured with mitomycin-treated pericytes were counted electronically. As expected, the number of pericytes was constant over the time course of the experiment. Thus, the data in Figure 1a present the changes in EC number only. The ECs cultured alone grew steadily over the 14-day time course, tripling in number. In contrast, the capillary ECs that were grown in the presence of the pericytes did not grow at all during the same time period, indicating a total inhibition of cell growth. Similar growth inhibition was observed when ECs were cocultured with aortic SMCs.

Coculture of ECs and Pericytes without Contact

To determine the role that contact or proximity between ECs and pericytes plays in the observed growth inhibition, ECs and pericytes were cocultured in a system that prevented contact between the two cell types but allowed free exchange of diffusible substances. This was accomplished by plating the mitomycin-treated pericytes into the bottom of multiwell dishes and the ECs into Millicell chambers, which are inserted into the wells. The Millicell chamber, lined by a porous membrane (0.45 μm) that makes exchange of soluble components possible, is held 1–2 mm above the pericyte layer. Under these culture conditions, no inhibition of EC growth was observed (Fig. 1b).

Effect of Other Cells on EC Growth

To assess the specificity of the observed pericyte inhibition of EC growth, retinal epithelial cells (RPE), fibroblasts, and 3T3 cells were examined for their ability to modulate EC growth. All three cell types were growth-arrested and cocultured directly with ECs as described for the EC-pericyte coculture experiments. None of these cells inhibited the growth of ECs. On the contrary, coculture of ECs with epithelial cells, fibroblasts, and 3T3 cells significantly stimulated EC proliferation to varying degrees with the stimulation of epithelial cells > 3T3 > fibroblasts.

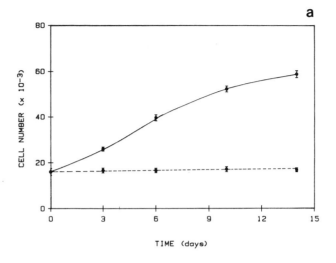

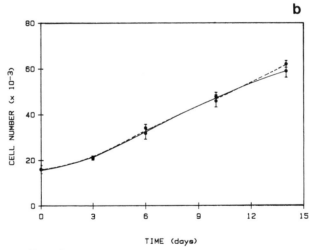

Figure 1 Effect of pericytes on capillary EC growth in cocultures. (*a*) With direct contact. Pericytes were growth-arrested with mitomycin C, plated into 24-well dishes, and allowed to attach overnight. An equal number of ECs were then plated into the wells containing the pericytes and into other wells alone. The change in EC number for cells cultured alone (—) and cocultured (directly) with pericytes (-----) was measured over 14 days. (*b*) Without contact. Pericytes were growth-arrested and plated as described above. In this case, an equal number of ECs were plated into Millicell inserts (Millipore), which allow for the exchange of diffusible molecules but prevent cell contact. The change in cell number of ECs cultured alone (—) and cocultured (without contact) with pericytes (-----) was measured over 14 days.

127

Effect of Cell Ratio on Pericyte-mediated Inhibition of EC Growth

To determine if alterations in the ratio of ECs to pericytes would influence the ability of pericytes to inhibit EC proliferation, ECs and pericytes were cocultured with direct contact at EC-to-pericyte ratios of 1:1, 2:1, 5:1, 10:1, and 20:1. EC proliferation was inhibited to the same extent at all ratios up to and including 10 ECs per 1 pericyte. At a ratio of 20 ECs per 1 pericyte, however, inhibition was observed only through day 6 of the time course. After that time, EC proliferation resumed and the cells grew at a rate similar to that of the controls, which were cultured alone.

Morphology

In cocultures at a ratio of 1:1, where contact between the cells was allowed, the ECs grew in discrete colonies whose perimeter was often defined by pericytes. ECs were never observed to overgrow the pericytes. In contrast, when ECs and RPE cells were cultured at a 1:1 ratio, the ECs never formed discrete colonies and appeared to freely overgrow the epithelial cells. At higher ratios, the pericytes were more scarce, and the ECs formed fewer colonies. Rather, pericytes were observed to extend more numerous processes, which appeared to contact neighboring ECs (Fig. 2).

DISCUSSION

Using cultures of capillary ECs and pericytes, we have tested the hypothesis that pericytes can suppress EC proliferation. By coculturing ECs and pericytes, we demonstrated that pericytes (and SMCs) can inhibit the growth of capillary ECs. Cocultures in which contact between the two cell types was prevented suggested that contact, or at least proximity, is required for the pericyte-mediated inhibition. Loss of the inhibition at higher EC-to-pericyte ratios and the observation of frequent contacts between the two cell types further support the idea that a physical interaction between pericytes and ECs is necessary for the inhibition.

A variety of clinical and experimental observations have indicated that the pericyte might act to suppress EC proliferation. For instance, prior to the retinal neovascularization in proliferative diabetic retinopathy, there is a phenomenon referred to as pericyte dropout, in which the retinal pericytes "degenerate" (Speiser et al. 1968). Similarly, ultrastructural observations of wound healing correlate the appearance of pericytes with the cessation of vessel growth (Crocker et al.

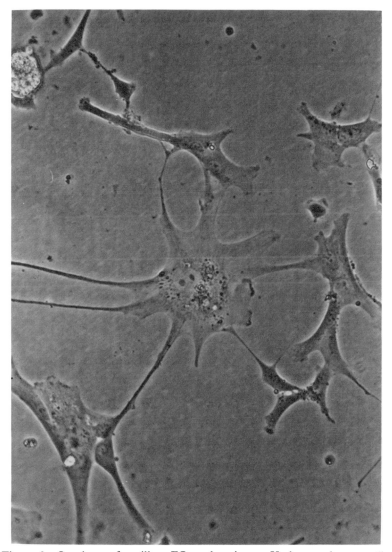

Figure 2 Coculture of capillary ECs and pericytes. Under coculture conditions, the pericyte (*center*) extends numerous processes, which appear to contact multiple ECs.

1970). However, because of technical difficulties involved in manipulating the pericyte in vivo, this possibility has gone unexamined. The experimental observations presented here strongly suggest that EC growth can be modulated by pericytes. Thus, cell-cell interactions may contribute to microvascular growth control.

REFERENCES

Crocker, D.J., T.M. Murad, and J.C. Geer. 1970. Role of the pericyte in wound healing. *Exp. Mol. Pathol.* **13**: 51.

Folkman, J., C.C. Haudenschild, and B.R. Zetter. 1979. Long-term culture of capillary endothelial cells. *Proc. Natl. Acad. Sci.* **76**: 5217.

Gitlin, J.D. and P.A. D'Amore. 1983. Culture of retinal capillary cells using selective growth media. *Microvasc. Res.* 26: 74.

Herman, I.M. and P.A. D'Amore. 1985. Microvascular pericytes contain muscle and nonmuscle actins. *J. Cell Biol.* **101**: 43.

Hobson, B. and J. Denekamp. 1984. Endothelial proliferation in tumours and normal tissue: Continuous labeling studies. *Br. J. Cancer* **49**: 405.

Speiser, P., A.M. Gittelsohn, and A. Patz. 1968. Studies on diabetic retinopathy. *Arch. Ophthalmol.* **80**: 332.

Differential Angiogenesis

R. Auerbach

Laboratory of Developmental Biology, Department of Zoology
University of Wisconsin, Madison, Wisconsin 53706

Angiogenesis, the formation of blood vessels, is a time- and site-specific process. Vascularization, both during normal development of the embryo and as an adjunct of pathological and reparative processes, does not occur indiscriminately. Rather, vessels are formed at a specific time and at a specific place in response to a variety of stimuli.

During embryogenesis, blood vessel formation occurs with precision, each organ establishing its unique capillaries and vascular connections as it differentiates from its early rudimentary anlage. The method by which this vasculogenesis is regulated in time and space is not yet understood. The methods by which the neovascular reactions that accompany wound healing, tumor growth, delayed hypersensitivity reactions, autoimmune reactions, and vasculitis are regulated are also not known.

HETEROGENEITY OF ENDOTHELIAL CELLS

The central hypothesis in our laboratory is that vascular endothelial cells are not all alike and that their differences reflect, in large part, their developmental origins (Auerbach and Joseph 1983). These differences have been documented by the use of immunological probes, by analysis of lectin-binding sites on the cell surface, and by assessment of adhesive interactions with tumor cells.

Organ-specific Antigens Expressed by Endothelial Cells

We have generated a panel of monoclonal antibodies directed against organ-specific cell-surface antigens. Using these antibodies, we have shown that organ-specific antigens are expressed on endothelial cells. For example, an antibody generated against rat ovary cells binds to mouse ovarian fibroblasts and endothelial cells derived from mouse ovary but fails to bind to fibroblasts or endothelial cells from other organs. Similarly, some brain-specific antibodies mark brain endothelial cells as well as neural cells selectively, whereas others define antigens unique to lung (Auerbach et al. 1985). Ia antigens are present on most endothelial cells, but not on brain-derived endothelial cells; Thy-1 is expressed on brain microvascular cells, but not on other endothelial cells.

Lectin-binding Properties of Endothelial Cells

We have recently isolated mouse endothelial cells from a variety of sites, including large vessel endothelial cells from aorta and thoracic duct, as well as microvascular cells from brain, liver, placenta, ovary, lung, retina, choroid, and epididymal fat pad. Of these, we compared aortic, thoracic duct, brain, lung, and liver endothelial cells with respect to their lectin-binding capacity (Gumkowski et al. 1987). Using a panel of seven lectins, we were able to demonstrate by flow cytometric analysis that each of these endothelial cell cultures manifested a unique lectin-binding profile. For example, brain and liver endothelial cells bound peanut agglutinin, in contrast to the other cells tested, but brain endothelial cells labeled tenfold more brightly than liver endothelial cells. On the other hand, thoracic duct and aortic endothelial cells labeled strongly with soybean agglutinin, but liver and lung endothelial cells were only marginally labeled. All endothelial cells tested bound ricin agglutinin, but liver endothelial cells labeled 12 times more brightly than brain endothelial cells.

Tumor Cell Adhesion to Endothelial Cell Monolayers

We have examined the relative efficiency by which different tumor cell types adhere to different endothelial cell monolayers (Alby and Auerbach 1984; Auerbach et al. 1987). Each tumor tested (S180 sarcoma; OTT-6050-derived teratoma; Hoak endothelioma, H7777 hepatoma, C755 mammary adenocarcinoma, MBT-2 bladder carcinoma, BW5147 lymphoma, GL26 glioma) behaved differently when tested on a panel of endothelial cells (aorta, lung, brain, liver, ovary) and fibroblasts (3T3, L929). Moreover, several of the tumors showed preferential adhesion to the endothelial cells corresponding to their in vivo affinity. Thus, the GL26 glioma adhered best to brain-derived endothelium, the ovary-seeking OTT-6050 teratoma to ovary-derived endothelium, the mammary tumor to lymphatic endothelium, and the H7777 hepatoma to liver-derived endothelial cells.

DISCUSSION

Studies of experimental angiogenesis have not addressed the question of selective neovascularization. Tests for angiogenesis (e.g., corneal assays, chorioallantoic membrane grafts, chemokinesis or proliferation of endothelial cells) have not been designed to detect differential vascular responses, nor are they likely to permit detection of fluctuations in production of, or responsiveness to, angiogenesis-inducing factors.

We suggest that the heterogeneity of endothelial cells that we have documented in our laboratory may provide the basis for time- and site-specific angiogenesis. For example, autoimmune-associated vascu-

132

larization may occur when angiogenic lymphokines are released by sensitized lymphocytes restimulated by organ-specific antigens present on endothelial cells (Watt and Auerbach 1986; Joseph et al. 1987). Similarly, tumor-derived angiogenesis factors may only be effective if released at sites where tumor cell adhesion to endothelium permits the establishment of gradients of these factors (Alby and Auerbach 1984; Auerbach et al. 1987), since such gradients may be essential for inducing the migration of vascular endothelial cells.

ACKNOWLEDGMENTS

The original research studies discussed in this paper have been carried out in collaboration with Marek Kaminski, Wei Cheng Lu, Grazyna Kaminska, Joanne Weber, Francine Gumkowski, Jeymohan Joseph, Louis Kubai, Jane Bielich, and Lawrence Morrissey. I am indebted to Wanda Auerbach for editorial assistance. These studies were supported, in part, by grants EY-3243 and CA-28656 from the National Institutes of Health and by grant PCM-3794 from the National Science Foundation.

REFERENCES

Alby, L. and R. Auerbach. 1984. Differential adhesion of tumor cells to capillary endothelial cells in vitro. *Proc. Natl. Acad. Sci.* **81:** 5739.

Auerbach, R. and J. Joseph. 1983. Cell surface markers on endothelial cells: A developmental perspective. In *The biology of endothelial cells* (ed. E.A. Jaffe), p. 393. Martinus Nijhoff, The Hague.

Auerbach, R., L. Alby, L.W. Morrissey, M. Tu, and J. Joseph. 1985. Expression of organ-specific antigens on capillary endothelial cells. *Microvasc. Res.* **29:** 401.

Auerbach, R., W.C. Lu, E. Pardon, F. Gumkowski, G. Kaminska, and M. Kaminski. 1987. Specificity of adhesion between tumor cells and capillary endothelium: An in vitro correlate of preferential metastasis in vivo. *Cancer Res.* **47:** (in press).

Gumkowski, F., G. Kaminska, M. Kaminski, L.W. Morrissey, and R. Auerbach. 1987. Heterogeneity of mouse vascular endothelium: In vitro studies of lymphatic large blood vessels and microvascular endothelial cells. *Blood Vessels* **24:** (in press).

Joseph, J., J.S. Cairns, and R. Auerbach. 1987. Ia antigens of murine epididymal fat pad endothelial cells. Immunohistology and mixed lymphocyte-endothelial cell culture studies. *Transplantation* **43:** (in press).

Watt, S.L. and R. Auerbach. 1986. A mitogenic factor for endothelial cells obtained from mouse secondary mixed leukocyte cultures. *J. Immunol.* **136:** 197.

Regulation of Embryonic Blood Vessel Development

W. Risau, R. Hallmann, H. Sariola, P. Ekblom, R. Kemler, and T. Doetschman

Max-Planck-Institut für Entwicklungsbiologie and
Friedrich-Miescher-Laboratorium der Max-Planck-Gesellschaft
D-7400 Tübingen, Federal Republic of Germany

The vascular system originates from blood islands that differentiate from the splanchnopleuric mesoderm of the area vasculosa. Blood islands consist of blood cell precursor cells in the center and immature endothelial cells at the periphery. They appear very early during embryogenesis. Blood islands grow, fuse, and form a primary capillary plexus. Outside the embryo, this capillary plexus gives rise to the yolk sac arteries, veins, and capillaries. Capillary plexae that have differentiated in situ in the embryo may fuse to become the aortic arches and dorsal aortas or may remain capillary plexae, which will give rise to new blood vessels (e.g., perineural vascular plexus, limb bud plexus). Although the basic morphological steps of the development of the vascular system have been described (for review, see Romanoff 1960), very little is known about the molecular mechanisms that stimulate angiogenesis. We have therefore used several experimental approaches and model systems to characterize the factors that regulate embryonic angiogenesis.

Embryonic Stem Cells

The early mammalian embryo is not amenable to in vitro investigations and manipulations. Embryonic stem cells (ESCs) have been established directly from the inner cell mass cells of mouse blastocysts (Doetschman et al. 1985). When kept on a feeder layer of embryonic fibroblasts, they proliferate but do not differentiate. After withdrawal from the feeder, they spontaneously differentiate in suspension culture through a series of embryoid bodies of increasing complexity, culminating in blood-island-containing visceral yolk-sac-like cystic embryoid bodies (Doetschman et al. 1985). The blood islands that form in vitro are morphologically indistinguishable from their in vivo counterparts. Figure 1 shows that blood islands derived from cystic embryoid bodies are capable of fusing and giving rise to capillaries when grown intraperitoneally.

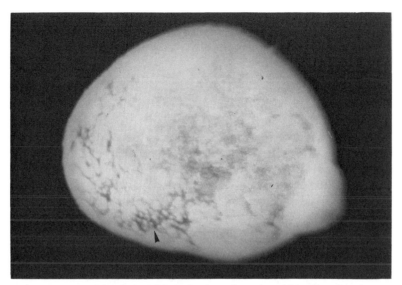

Figure 1 Blood islands in ESC-derived cystic embryoid bodies give rise to a capillary plexus (arrowhead) when injected intraperitoneally into mice.

The incidence of blood island development in vitro is, however, dependent on the culture conditions. Human cord serum, instead of fetal bovine serum, greatly enhanced the development of blood islands, whereas purified growth factors (e.g., epidermal growth factor and fibroblast growth factor) and hemopoietic factors had no such dramatic effect. Extracts from 10-day mouse embryos could also stimulate the development of blood islands in vitro. We do not know at present which human cord serum factors are responsible for this effect, but our in vitro system may allow us to isolate and characterize them. Such factors might be involved in the induction of blood islands and/or hemopoiesis.

Transplantation of ESC-derived complex and cystic embryoid bodies onto the quail chorioallantoic membrane (CAM) showed that CAM blood vessels were attracted by these cells. This response, however, was directed by the differentiated non-yolk-sac endoderm structures found within the embryoid bodies and not by the yolk sac endoderm. This is consistent with our results showing that embryonic yolk sac dissected from an embryo will not give rise to an angiogenic response when transplanted onto a CAM. Since embryoid bodies at the cyst formation stage (about 10 days of suspension culture) show the highest angiogenic response on the quail CAM, they have been used to isolate and characterize an angiogenic factor that is similar to fibroblast growth factor according to biochemical criteria (heparin-Sepharose chromatography). Our results indicate that differentiated embryonic stem cells are a good in vitro model system to study early blood vessel development.

Embryonic Brain Angiogenesis

The neural tube does not contain any blood vessels early in embryonic development but is surrounded by a primitive perineural vascular plexus (Evans 1909). From here, capillaries invade neural tissue at a defined time of development that correlates well with the onset of neural ectodermal proliferation.

By using the chick-quail nuclear marking technique developed by LeDouarin (1973), Stewart and Wiley (1981) showed that brain capillaries are indeed derived from outside blood vessels. We have recently isolated and characterized an angiogenesis factor from embryonic chick brain. This factor is a heparin-binding endothelial cell growth factor of about 16 kD and is therefore similar to the well-characterized fibroblast growth factors. Its specific activity is high in the early embryonic brain (Risau 1986).

Embryonic Kidney Angiogenesis

Embryonic kidneys induce angiogenesis when transplanted onto the quail CAM. All blood vessels in these transplants were derived from the quail host (Ekblom et al. 1982). Interestingly, only embryonic kidneys containing the ureter bud, which in vivo induces the differentiation of the nephrogenic mesenchyme into kidney epithelial cells, induce angiogenesis in vivo on the CAM or in the rabbit cornea. Embryonic mouse kidneys produce a heparin-binding angiogenic endothelial cell growth factor of 18 kD (Risau and Ekblom 1986). The differentiation-dependent production of an angiogenesis factor by the embryonic kidney suggests an important role of angiogenesis in organogenesis.

Angiogenesis and Endothelial Cell Differentiation

It is important to keep in mind that capillaries not only serve as a pipeline for nutrient and oxygen delivery, but have various other functions in different organs. Brain capillaries, for example, form the blood-brain barrier, and glomerular capillaries in the kidney are the site of blood filtration. It is not known how the differentiation of these endothelial cells, which are derived from outside blood vessels, is regulated. Preliminary evidence suggests that the interaction between endothelial cells and the special tissue environment plays a major role (Stewart and Wiley 1981; Risau et al. 1986).

Embryonic versus Adult Angiogenesis
The detection of angiogenesis factors in embryonic organs known to stimulate blood vessel ingrowth at a well-defined developmental stage suggests that these factors have a function in embryonic development. Endothelium in adult tissues has a very low turnover (Denekamp 1984). There is normally no active vascularization process in adult tissues, except for ovulation and corpus luteum formation. Nevertheless, considerable amounts of endothelial cell growth factors have been found in adult tissues, particularly in the brain and kidney. Recent evidence suggests that these factors are not newly synthesized but are stored in adult tissues (Abraham et al. 1986). It is unclear how they are kept in an inactive form.

Regression of Blood Vessels
During embryogenesis, the vascular system rapidly develops but is also constantly remodeled. Remodeling involves regression of major parts of the vascular system (e.g., yolk sac), but also of defined blood vessels, such as aortic arches.

An interesting phenomenon of a local predetermined regression of capillaries occurs during limb morphogenesis. Capillaries in the skeletal anlagen of the limb regress in a characteristic spatial and temporal pattern (Feinberg et al. 1986). We have analyzed the regression of capillaries and the differentiation of cartilage in limb bud sections using fluorescent acetylated low-density lipoprotein as a marker for capillaries and a monoclonal antibody against cartilage. Our results show that capillaries actually regress before cartilage differentiates (R. Hallmann et al., in prep.).

CONCLUDING REMARKS
Embryonic stem cells, embryonic neural tissues, and the embryonic kidney are all strong stimulators of angiogenesis. We have found that all these tissues contain heparin-binding angiogenesis factors. We postulate that these factors, at least in part, regulate the initiation of angiogenesis.

In the embryo, a rapid regression of capillaries also takes place. Interestingly, in the developing limb bud, a controlled local regression occurs while the rest of the limb vasculature is still growing. It is likely that as yet unidentified inhibitory factors are crucial for this process.

REFERENCES
Abraham, J.A., J.L. Whang, A. Tumolo, A. Mergia, J. Friedman, D. Gospodarowicz, and J.C. Fiddes. 1986. Human basic fibroblast growth factor: Nucleotide sequence and genomic organization. *EMBO J*. 5: 2523.

Denekamp, J. 1984. Vascular endothelium as the vulnerable element in tumours. *Acta Radiol. Oncol.* **23**: 217.

Doetschman, T.C., H. Eistetter, M. Katz, W. Schmidt, and R. Kemler. 1985. The in vitro development of blastocyst-derived embryonic stem cell lines: Formation of visceral yolk sac, blood islands and myocardium. *J. Embryol. Exp. Morphol.* **87**: 27.

Ekblom, P., H. Sariola, M. Karkinen, and L. Saxén. 1982. The origin of the glomerular endothelium. *Cell Differ.* **11**: 35.

Evans, H.M. 1909. On the development of the aortae, cardinal and umbilical veins, and the other blood vessels of vertebrate embryos from capillaries. *Anat. Rec.* **3**: 498.

Feinberg, R.N., C.H. Latker, and D.C. Beebe. 1986. Localized vascular regression during limb morphogenesis in the chicken embryo. I. Spatial and temporal changes in the vascular pattern. *Anat. Rec.* **214**: 405.

LeDouarin, N. 1973. A biological cell labeling technique and its use in experimental embryology. *Dev. Biol.* **30**: 217.

Risau, W. 1986. Developing brain produces an angiogenesis factor. *Proc. Natl. Acad. Sci.* **83**: 3855.

Risau, W. and P. Ekblom. 1986. Production of a heparin-binding angiogenesis factor by the embryonic kidney. *J. Cell Biol.* **103**: 1101.

Risau, W., R. Hallmann, U. Albrecht, and S. Henke-Fahle. 1986. Brain induces the expression of an early cell surface marker for blood-brain barrier specific endothelium. *EMBO J.* **5**: 3179.

Romanoff, A.L. 1960. *The avian embryo.* Macmillan Company, New York.

Stewart, P.A. and M.J. Wiley. 1981. Developing nervous tissue induces formation of blood-brain barrier characteristics in invading endothelial cells: A study using quail-chick transplantation chimeras. *Dev. Biol.* **84**: 183.

Proliferation and Migration of Irradiated Endothelial Cells

M.M. Sholley and J.D. Wilson

Departments of Anatomy and Radiology, Medical College of Virginia
Virginia Commonwealth University, Richmond, Virginia 23298

In this paper, we describe the radiation survival characteristics of endothelial cells (ECs) during angiogenesis in vivo and during colony formation in vitro. For cycling cells, the radiobiological definition of survival is the ability of a cell to proliferate indefinitely following irradiation. Operationally, survival is usually measured in vitro using colony formation assays, which are based on the ability of individual surviving cells to form clones and allow construction of standard log-linear survival curves. For radiation such as X rays, survival curves for mammalian cells typically have a shoulder region at low doses and an exponential region at higher doses. Parameters used to describe such curves include D_o, which is the dose increment that reduces survival by the factor 0.37 on the exponential portion of the curve and is taken as a measure of radiosensitivity, and n, which is the back-extrapolated y-intercept of the exponential part of the curve and is a measure of shoulder width. Similar curves may be plotted using dose-response data from in vivo studies, but indirect assessment of cellular survival based on various measurements of growth may be influenced by factors other than clonogenicity of the cells. Nevertheless, important information regarding the effects of radiation on angiogenesis and information on the cellular mechanisms underlying formation of new vessels may be obtained by in vivo studies.

MECHANISMS OF ANGIOGENESIS FOLLOWING IRRADIATION

Our previous studies of mechanisms of angiogenesis in the rat cornea have shown that initial vascular growth is a very radioresistant process (Sholley et al. 1984). In corneas exposed to high single doses (2000–8000 rads) of X rays immediately prior to central cauterization using silver nitrate, vascular sprouting at 2 days was comparable to the results in shielded controls, and formation of new vessels continued until 4 days. [³H]Thymidine autoradiography demonstrated that proliferation

139

of ECs was prevented by the high radiation doses, and ultrastructural analysis indicated that the nonproliferative vascular growth resulted from migration and elongation of ECs from the limbal vessels. This radioresistant vascular growth is represented by the second components of biphasic dose-response curves based on length of vascular penetration at 4 days and 7 days. The second components at both 4 days and 7 days are represented on a linear plot by the same gradually sloping straight line, indicating that radioresistant growth did not continue after 4 days. Log-linear plots of normalized length data at 4 days and 7 days display common initial slopes, breakpoints at about 1200 and 2000 rads, respectively, and resistant tails having identical slopes. Back-extrapolation of the radioresistant components to zero dose suggests that they accounted for 70% of total length at 4 days and 40% at 7 days. Thus, migration of existing cells contributes less to the total growth as length increases, and cellular proliferation becomes essential for continuation of angiogenesis. The effect of radiation on cellular proliferation is reflected on the dose-response curves by the common initial components, which have a steeper slope than the second components, demonstrating that proliferation of ECs is a more radiosensitive process than cellular migration and elongation.

Survival of Irradiated Endothelial Cells In Vivo

To assess proliferative survival of ECs during angiogenesis in the cornea, dose-response curves based on vascular length were adjusted by subtracting the contribution of the migratory growth mechanism. Since proliferation accounts for a higher percentage of total growth in longer assays, only 7-day vascular length data were used for this analysis. Figure 1 illustrates the radiosensitive component at doses between 500 and 2000 rads in both unadjusted and adjusted forms. Adjustment was performed by back-extrapolating the radioresistant component on the original (linear plot) dose-response curves, subtracting this resistant length from the total length, and then normalizing the data for plotting in log-linear form. At a dose of 500 rads, both curves in Figure 1 demonstrate that vascular length was unaffected, suggesting that proliferation was not decreased. However, it is possible that proliferating cells were lost, but that vascular length as an endpoint is not sensitive enough to reflect loss of small numbers of cells. On the other hand, [^{3}H]thymidine autoradiographic studies following exposure to 500 rads demonstrated that endothelial DNA synthesis was significantly inhibited only at 1 day after irradiation, having recovered by 2 days, exceeded control levels at 4 days, and matched control levels at 7 days. The unadjusted and adjusted curves are exponential at doses above

1000 rads and have D_o values of 1250 and 245 rads, respectively, the latter number representing the radiosensitivity of endothelial proliferation without migration.

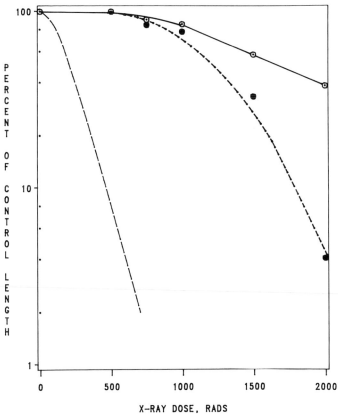

Figure 1 Radiation dose-response of angiogenesis in the rat cornea. Immediately following X-irradiation of the left cornea, angiogenesis was induced in both corneas of each animal by standardized central cauterization with silver nitrate. The length of penetration of new vessels was measured following colloidal carbon perfusion at 7 days. The mean length in unirradiated corneas was 1.92 mm. Only the initial component of the resulting biphasic dose-response curve is plotted. (○) Plot of normalized total growth, representing the contributions of both migration and proliferation of ECs; (●) plot of normalized adjusted growth, representing the contribution of proliferation alone. The curves were determined by fitting the experimental data to a multitarget, single-hit model using a nonlinear regression procedure. The D_o values are 1250 rads for the total growth and 245 rads for the adjusted growth. (-----) In vitro clonogenic response of HUVECs, plotted for comparison with the in vivo curves.

Survival of Irradiated Endothelial Cells In Vitro

We studied in vitro survival of human umbilical vein endothelial cells (HUVECs) using a colony formation assay. To our knowledge, colony formation assays have not previously been used to study the survival of HUVECs. HUVECs were grown in gelatin-coated flasks in medium supplemented with fetal bovine serum, endothelial cell growth factor (ECGF), and heparin. Confluent HUVECs in the fifth or sixth passage were trypsinized and replated at a density of 1000 or 10,000 cells per T-25 flask. Irradiation was performed 20 hours later and colonies were counted after 10–13 days. The resulting survival curve, shown in Figure 2, had a D_0 of 146 rads and an n of 2.4. Although colony formation is the preferred assay, we also used an in vitro growth assay for comparison. Confluent first passage HUVECs were irradiated and then replated at a density of 125,000 cells per T-25 flask. Total cell number was assessed after 7 days of growth. As shown in Figure 2, the survival curve based on growth inhibition was similar to that obtained with the colony formation assay. It had a D_0 of 132 rads and an n of 2.6. DeGowin et al. (1976) also used growth assays to study the radiation response of HUVECs, but without ECGF and heparin. They found a D_0 of 160 rads. All of the values for D_0 in these studies of HUVECs are similar, suggesting that there are no differences in the radiosensitivities determined by the two methods. The D_0 values obtained from colony formation assays with ECs from bovine arteries (161 rads, Kwock et al. 1982; 101 rads, Rhee et al. 1986) and rabbit aortas (120 rads, Martin and Fischer 1984) were similar to those for HUVECs.

Comparison of Endothelial Radiosensitivity In Vivo and In Vitro

Values for D_0 determined from in vitro assays of endothelial clonogenicity and growth are much lower than those determined from in vivo assays of angiogenesis (compare the in vitro and in vivo curves plotted together in Fig. 1). This difference may mean that ECs in vivo are less radiosensitive or it may reflect differences in the biological endpoints measured in vitro versus in vivo. Mechanisms not dependent on cellular survival could contribute to vascular length in vivo. For example, by increasing their surface areas, a smaller number of surviving ECs in an irradiated cornea might produce the same vascular length as a larger number of cells in an unirradiated cornea. Also, irradiated cells that cannot proliferate or that can undergo only a limited number of divisions might contribute to vascular length.

The shoulders of the in vitro survival curves are much smaller than those of the in vivo curves. Note in Figure 2 that at 500 rads the in vitro curve is already exponential and the surviving fraction has been reduced to about 0.08, whereas the in vivo response has not been

142

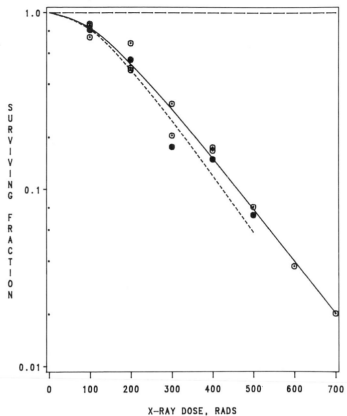

Figure 2 Radiation dose-response curves of HUVECs in vitro. The curves were determined by fitting the experimental data to a multitarget, single-hit model using a nonlinear regression procedure. (○) Survival of ECs determined by colony formation assay; D_o is 146 rads and the n is 2.4. (●) Inhibition of proliferation in a 7-day growth assay; D_o is 132 rads and the n is 2.6. (-----) Adjusted response of angiogenesis in vivo, plotted for comparison with the in vitro curves.

reduced. The wider shoulder could indicate a greater capacity of ECs to accumulate and/or repair radiation damage under the in vivo conditions, which allowed an interval between immediate postirradiation cauterization and actual stimulation of the limbal vessels by diffusing chemical products. Indeed, when the radiation was delivered 6 hours after silver nitrate cauterization, allowing less time for quiescent cells to repair radiation damage before actual stimulation, the shoulder was reduced as was the D_o. It is difficult in vitro to model the situation in which normal vessels are irradiated prior to stimulation, because even confluent endothelial cultures have higher percentages of proliferating cells than unstimulated vessels in vivo. Our in vivo experiments, then, may represent optimal conditions for survival of irradiated ECs: irradiation of quiescent cells with time for repair of radiation damage before stimulation.

DISCUSSION

It should be noted that our in vivo assay involved microvascular ECs and the in vitro assays involved ECs from large vessels. There also were species differences. It remains to be determined whether ECs from small and large vessels of the same species would have the same survival characteristics in clonogenic assays in vitro. Concerning the available data on the radiosensitivity of ECs, it seems that the in vitro data are the least complicated and the most amenable for comparison to data concerning other cell types measured in vitro. However, because the radiosensitivity of angiogenesis as a process is less than would be predicted from the in vitro data on survival of ECs, the in vivo studies may provide a more clinically relevant endpoint in terms of the response of intact tissues to radiation.

ACKNOWLEDGMENTS

The authors thank Ms. Megan Borror, Mr. Stephen Gudas, and Ms. Gilda Ferguson for excellent technical assistance. This work was supported in part by grant CA-26316 from the National Cancer Institute, Department of Health and Human Services.

REFERENCES

DeGowin, R.L., L.J. Lewis, R.E. Mason, M.K. Borke, and J.C. Hoak. 1976. Radiation-induced inhibition of human endothelial cells replicating in culture. *Radiat. Res.* **68**: 244.

Kwock, L., W.H.J. Douglas, P.S. Lin, W.E. Baur, and B.L. Fanburg. 1982. Endothelial cell damage after gamma-irradiation in vitro: Impaired uptake of alpha-aminoisobutyric acid. *Am. Rev. Respir. Dis.* **125**: 95.

Martin, D.F. and J.J. Fischer. 1984. Radiation sensitivity of cultured rabbit aortic endothelial cells. *Int. J. Radiat. Oncology Biol. Phys.* **10**: 1903.

Rhee, J.G., I. Lee, and C.W. Song. 1986. The clonogenic response of bovine aortic endothelial cells in culture to radiation. *Radiat. Res.* **106**: 182.

Sholley, M.M., G.P. Ferguson, H.R. Seibel, J.L. Montour, and J.D. Wilson. 1984. Mechanisms of neovascularization: Vascular sprouting can occur without proliferation of endothelial cells. *Lab. Invest.* **51**: 624.

Growth Factors Recruit Cells and Modulate Collagen Degradation in Wound Repair and Human Skin Fibroblasts

J.M. Davidson, A. Buckley, S.C. Woodward, R.M. Senior,* G.L. Griffin,* and M. Klagsbrun†

Department of Pathology
Vanderbilt University School of Medicine and Research Service
VA Medical Center, Nashville, Tennessee 37203

*Respiratory and Critical Care Division, Department of Medicine
Jewish Hospital at Washington University Medical Center
St. Louis, Missouri 63110

†Departments of Biological Chemistry and Surgery
The Children's Hospital and Harvard Medical School
Boston, Massachusetts 07215

Wound repair is a complex process involving the progressive infiltration of inflammatory cells, fibroblasts, and endothelial cells into the wound site, followed by the remodeling of granulation tissue into a functional extracellular matrix. The success and rate of the process can be measured by collagen accumulation, which can be equated to tissue strength, and the formation of new blood vessels. Both inflammatory and mesenchymal cells possess the capacity to produce and secrete cellular growth factors that may mediate or accelerate the repair process. A model system, the polyvinyl alcohol sponge implanted subcutaneously in 200-g rats, has been used to evaluate the hypothesis that growth factors can affect the rate of wound repair. Previous studies show that a species of basic fibroblast growth factor (bFGF) derived from bovine cartilage (cartilage-derived growth factor [CDGF]) (Davidson et al. 1985; Sullivan and Klagsbrun 1985) and epidermal growth factor (EGF) (Buckley et al. 1985) are capable of accelerating the rate of formation of collagen, DNA, and capillaries in experimental granulation tissue. Preliminary evidence has suggested that at least CDGF is not acting simply as a mitogen, since recruitment of cells to the wound site appears to play an important role in increasing cell number. The present studies were aimed at comparing the specific mechanisms by which such growth factors influence repair at wound sites. Two activities related to cell movement and tissue reorganization were considered: chemotaxis and the production of latent collagenase.

145

RESULTS

Initial experiments showed that CDGF was a potent chemoattractant. Using ligamentum nuchae fibroblasts (provided by R.P. Mecham) as a standardized target, maximal effects on directed cell movement were obtained at 1 ng/ml (approx. 50 pM). Comparable results were obtained with a related cationic growth factor isolated from chondrosarcoma by heparin-affinity chromatography (ChDGF) (Shing et al. 1984). Checkerboard assays showed that (1) both factors evoked specific chemoattraction rather than chemokinesis, and (2) CDGF and ChDGF, at equivalent concentrations, competed for cell movement. These results strengthened the role of CDGF in fibroblast recruitment.

To demonstrate that cells specifically involved in wound repair responded to these factors, granulation tissue fibroblasts were isolated from sponge granulomas at various stages in the repair process. Primary cultures, containing a mixed population of cells, were passaged once to produce uniformly fibroblastic cultures. Populations from d6, d14, and d28 sponges were evaluated, representing stages of rapid cellular infiltration, reorganization of tissue matrix, and terminal differentiation. Platelet-derived growth factor (PDGF; kindly supplied by T. Deuel) was used as a positive control for chemotaxis in the Boyden-chamber assay. Although granulation tissue fibroblasts from all stages of the repair process were stimulated to move toward CDGF, chemotactic responses were highest in the 14-day tissue and were significantly attenuated in cells from the 28-day tissue (Table 1). In contrast, all cells showed similar mitogenic responses. Epidermal growth factor (EGF) was highly chemotactic for both granulation tissue and human skin fibroblasts. Cells from all stages of sponge organization showed similar-

Table 1 Assay of Chemotactic Activity of Growth Factors

	Growth factor		
Cellular source	PDGF	EGF	CDGF
Day 6	30(10)	60(10)	46(1)
Day 14	42(10)	55(50)	34(0.1)
Day 28	43(10)	50(10)	19(1)
Human skin	25(10)	41(10)	n.d.

Granulation tissue cells explanted from sponges on the indicated days were assayed as secondary cultures in Boyden chambers. Data are expressed as cells per high-power field and represent the mean of five determinations in three chambers; s.e.m. < 10%. Numbers in parentheses indicate the dose, in ng/ml, giving the highest chemotactic response on a given cell population.

146

ly high levels of chemotactic activity toward EGF. On a molar basis, cells were 150–300 times more sensitive to CDGF and ChDGF, but EGF brought about more cell movement.

Remodeling of collagen is likely to be involved in cell movement, and it is certainly necessary for the reorganization of granulation tissue after cellular infiltration is complete. A sensitive assay for production of latent collagenase, using soluble [^{3}H]collagen, was used to quantify the effects of CDGF and EGF on production of the enzyme. Granulation tissue fibroblasts showed considerable variation in the production of latent collagenase, depending on cell density and population heterogeneity. Only secondary cultures of confluent granulation tissue fibroblasts that had been cultured in serum (acid-treated) produced significant quantities of the latent enzyme, and production was low unless stimulated by factors such as phorbol myristic acid (PMA) or interleukin-1.

Unlike the similarities found in chemotactic activity of CDGF and EGF, these two growth factors were distinctly different with respect to collagenase production in this cell population (Fig. 1). Cells from d6 sponges showed clear dose responses to 8–64 ng/ml of CDGF, whereas EGF had no effect whatsoever on enzyme release at doses up to 640 ng/ml. Fibroblasts from fully organized (d21) sponges were not responsive to CDGF, EGF, or PMA, yet all of the cell populations showed positive mitogenic responses to each of the growth factors.

Human skin fibroblasts were also responsive to CDGF and ChDGF. Doses up to 64 ng/ml stimulated constitutive production of latent collagenase activity three- to fourfold. In addition, the response was not attenuated in fibroblasts derived from older skin (70 years).

DISCUSSION

Growth factors are conventionally described by their capacity to stimulate cells to divide under defined in vitro conditions. Their effects in vivo are less completely described. Although either injection of CDGF (a form of bFGF) or slow release of encapsulated EGF at the wound site stimulates angiogenesis, collagen accumulation, and other parameters of wound repair, the present results indicate important mechanistic differences. Both factors had the capacity to recruit directly mesenchymal cells to sites of wound repair. This appears to be a novel finding, for EGF at least. In contrast, EGF was not able to stimulate directly the production of a latent form of collagenase, an enzyme strongly implicated in wound repair (Grillo and Gross 1967) and angiogenesis (this volume). Other growth conditions may permit EGF responsiveness (Chua et al. 1985).

During the repair process, there appeared to be considerable changes

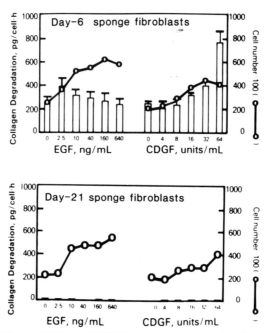

Figure 1 Effect of EGF and CDGF on mitogenesis and collagenase production in day-6 and day-21 granulation tissue fibroblasts. Cells were derived from experimental granulation tissue in 200-g rats at 6 days (*top*) and 21 days (*bottom*) after implantation. Activities were determined in secondary cultures. Varying doses of EGF (0–640 ng/ml) and CDGF (0–64 units/ml) were tested. One unit of CDGF causes half-maximal stimulation of 3T3 cell DNA synthesis and is equivalent to 1 ng of protein in homogeneous preparations. Mitogenesis was tested on subconfluent cells, and latent collagenase was measured in confluent cultures. Data represent the mean of four flasks assayed in triplicate ± S.E.M.

in the phenotype of the fibroblast population present within experimental granulation tissue, at least among those cells that could be propagated in culture. It is not known whether the morphologically mixed population of cells in primary cultures contained cells that suppressed the production of latent collagenase or whether further cell division was necessary to produce the response. Since all collagenase activity was latent, it remains to be determined what fraction of this enzyme is activated in situ during wound repair and to what extent inhibitors of collagenase may suppress the activated enzyme.

CDGF and EGF shared the common capacity to elicit directed cell movement but strongly differed in their ability to evoke at least one protease. If collagenase activity is indeed a prerequisite for reorganization of granulation tissue, EGF may have invoked a secondary signal in another cellular target within granulation tissue. CDGF was capable of stimulating both chemotaxis and collagenase production at similar, low molar concentrations, suggesting that the effects were mediated by high-affinity receptors. The differential chemotactic responsiveness of granulation tissue cells at different stages of the repair process could have represented a change in the efficiency of part of the signal transduction pathway. The chemotactic and mitogenic responses of PDGF are likewise distinguishable.

These results were consistent with the concept that either cell recruitment or tissue remodeling by proteases may be rate-limiting during the repair process. Further experimentation might indicate which growth factors and mechanisms are more essential to wound healing, particularly when it is compromised by conditions such as aging and the diabetic state.

ACKNOWLEDGMENTS

This work was supported, in part, by the Veterans Administration and by grants from the National Institutes of Health (AG-06528, HL-29594, and CA-21763).

REFERENCES

Buckley, A., J.M. Davidson, C.D. Kamerath, T.B. Wolt, and S.C. Woodward. 1985. Sustained release of epidermal growth factor accelerates wound repair. *Proc. Natl. Acad. Sci.* **82**: 7340.

Chua, C.-C., D.E. Geiman, E.H. Keller, and R.L. Ladda. 1985. Induction of collagenase secretion in human fibroblast cultures by growth promoting factors. *J. Biol. Chem.* **260**: 5213.

Davidson, J.M., M. Klagsbrun, K.E. Hill, A. Buckley, R. Sullivan, P.S. Brewer, and S.C. Woodward. 1985. Accelerated wound repair, cell proliferation, and collagen accumulation are produced by a cartilage-derived growth factor. *J. Cell Biol.* **100**: 1219.

Grillo, H.C. and J. Gross. 1967. Collagenolytic activity during mammalian wound repair. *Dev. Biol.* **15**: 300.

Shing, Y., J. Folkman, R. Sullivan, C. Butterfield, J. Murray, and M. Klagsbrun. 1984. Heparin affinity: Purification of a tumor-derived capillary endothelial cell growth factor. *Science* **223**: 1296.

Sullivan, R. and M. Klagsbrun. 1985. Purification of cartilage-derived growth factor by heparin affinity chromatography. *J. Biol. Chem.* **260**: 10115

Environmental Regulation of Macrophage Angiogenesis

D. Knighton, S. Schumerth, and V. Fiegel

Wound Healing Clinic and Laboratory, Department of Surgery
University of Minnesota, Minneapolis Veterans Administration
Minneapolis, Minnesota 55455

Most in vivo biologic or pathologic systems where angiogenesis occurs are associated with the presence of a local oxygen gradient created by high tissue metabolic demand, interruption of normal blood flow, or decrease in oxygen delivery. There are many examples. Malignant neoplasms (Brem et al. 1972; Folkman 1974), the corpus luteum (Gospodarowicz and Thakral 1977; Jakob et al. 1977), and chronic electrical stimulation of muscle (Hudlicka et al. 1977) produce local tissue hypoxia by high metabolic demand. Chronic ischemic tissue resulting from atherosclerosis (Makitie 1977; Hammarsten et al. 1980) and hypoxia associated with living at high altitudes (Valdivia 1958) produce local tissue hypoxia by interruption of normal blood flow or reduced FiO_2. The healing wound produces local tissue hypoxia by mechanical production of a hypoxic wound space and offers a unique experimental situation to study the relationship between local tissue hypoxia and the regulation of angiogenesis. Using a modification of Clark's rabbit ear wound chamber (Knighton et al. 1981), which allows manipulation of the central wound space pO_2, we demonstrated that a hypoxic wound space was required for normal wound-healing angiogenesis to occur. When the pO_2 was artificially raised above 100 mm Hg, neovascularization stopped, the capillary network matured, and the wound space remained avascular. This effect was reversible and occurred whether 15%, 30%, 60%, or 70% of the chamber was filled with new vessels (Knighton et al. 1981). These experiments demonstrated that a hypoxic central wound space was required for normal wound-healing angiogenesis to occur.

The mechanism by which changes in the local oxygen tension affect wound-healing angiogenesis was still in question. The only cells that populate the hypoxic, acidotic, hypercarbic, hypokalemic, hypoglycemic, hyperlactic wound space are neutrophils from wounding to day 3 and macrophages from day 3 to the end of repair (Hunt et al. 1981). Previous data showed that macrophages produce angiogenesis in various experimental systems (Polverini et al. 1977; Greenberg and

150

Hunt 1978; Thakral et al. 1979). To determine whether the wound macrophage is responsive to local changes in oxygen tension, rabbit bone marrow macrophages were exposed to various local oxygen tensions in culture and the supernatant was tested for angiogenesis, plasminogen activator (PA), and mitogenesis growth factor [GF]). Hypoxic (15 mm Hg) macrophages produced angiogenesis factor (AF) and PA activity, whereas hyperoxic (150 mm Hg) macrophages produced no AF or PA activity. GF activity was not affected by changes in pO_2. A dose-response curve was examined by culturing macrophages at 15, 40, 75, and 150 mm Hg. Cells kept at 15 mm Hg produced maximal AF activity (Fig. 1), those at 40 mm Hg produced a small amount of AF activity, and those at 75 and 150 mm Hg produced no AF activity. All other culture conditions were held at physiologic parameters (Knighton et al. 1983).

ROLE OF pH AND pO_2

To test whether pH also played a role in macrophage AF production, similar experiments were carried out at pH 6.0, 6.5, 7.0, 7.5, and 8.0. The results are summarized in Table 1. A positive angiogenesis assay reflects a rabbit corneal assay with a +2 rating or greater. Mitogenesis

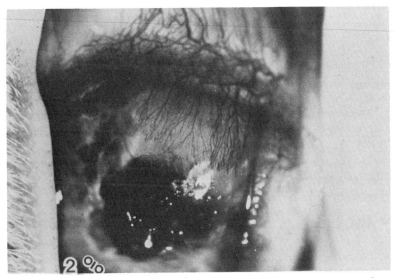

Figure 1 Hypoxic macrophage angiogenesis in the rabbit corneal assay. Conditioned medium was suspended in hydron polymer pellets and implanted into the cornea. Histology showed neovascularization with accompanying inflammation.

151

Table 1 Effect of pH and pO_2 on Macrophage Angiogenesis, Growth Factor, and Lactate

pO_2	pH	AF (+ tests/tot)	GF ($\pm$ s.d.)	Lactate (m M/l $\pm$ s.d.)
15	6.0	2/7	0.6 (0.3)	0.42 (0.01)
15	6.5	6/8	0.8 (0.3)	0.45 (0.04)
15	7.0	4/8	0.5 (0.5)	0.48 (0.01)
15	7.5	2/8	1.1 (0.5)	0.52 (0.10)
15	8.0	3/7	0.7 (0.3)	0.42 (0.08)
40	6.0	2/5	1.3 (0.5)	0.40 (0.03)
40	6.5	2/6	0.6 (0.4)	0.49 (0.05)
40	7.0	1/8	1.4 (0.6)	0.44 (0.04)
40	7.5	3/6	1.0 (0.7)	0.46 (0.04)
40	8.0	1/6	1.3 (0.6)	0.51 (0.05)
75	6.0	2/6	0.8 (0.3)	0.43 (0.05)
75	6.5	4/5	1.3 (0.7)	0.59 (0.16)
75	7.0	2/6	1.3 (0.4)	0.42 (0.08)
75	7.5	2/5	1.1 (0.8)	0.48 (0.06)
75	8.0	2/6	1.3 (0.5)	0.45 (0.03)
150	6.0	0/7	1.4 (0.8)	0.43 (0.05)
150	6.5	0/2	1.2 (0.7)	0.50 (0.07)
150	7.0	0/4	1.2 (0.5)	0.44 (0.08)
150	7.5	0/4	0.5 (0.2)	0.46 (0.00)
150	8.0	0/4	1.3 (0.8)	0.45 (0.06)

was measured on BALB/c-3T3 cells and is expressed as a mitogenic index, and lactate production was measured by standard laboratory methods.

The data confirm our prior observations that macrophages cultured at high oxygen tensions produce no angiogenesis activity regardless of the pH. At intermediate oxygen tension, there is a small amount of AF produced, and at 15 mm Hg, the greatest amount of AF activity was found at pH 6.5. These two environmental parameters correspond to those measured in the avascular wound space.

DISCUSSION

The results of these experiments also support a possible unifying mechanism for the regulation of angiogenesis in vivo. A focus of local tissue hypoxia, regardless of the cause, could stimulate a recruited or local tissue macrophage population to produce AF. As long as the hypoxic focus persists, macrophage AF production continues, producing neovascularization. When the physiologic or pathologic condition

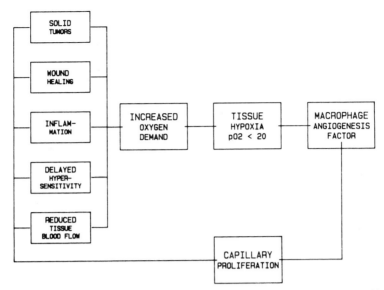

Figure 2 Proposed mechanism for macrophage environmental control of in vivo angiogenesis.

that produced the local tissue hypoxia is changed or corrected, normal tissue oxygen tension is reestablished, shutting off macrophage production of AF and the neovascularization process (Fig. 2).

To use the healing wound as an example, the creation of the wound space mechanically produces a hypoxic environment that is populated by macrophages. These cells produce AF and GF, which causes a vascularized collagen fibroblast mesh to fill the wound. When the two edges of the wound finally meet, the local hypoxic space is obliterated, raising the pO_2 above the threshold level for macrophage production of AF. This shuts off the signal for continued capillary growth, and the microvasculature matures into stable scar tissue.

REFERENCES

Brem, S., R. Cotran, and J. Folkman. 1972. Tumor angiogenesis: A quantitative method for histologic grading. *J. Natl. Cancer Inst.* **48**: 347.

Folkman, J. 1974. Tumor angiogenesis. *Adv. Cancer Res.* **10**: 331.

Gospodarowicz, D. and K.K. Thakral. 1977. Production of a corpus luteum angiogenic factor responsible for proliferation of capillaries and neovascularization of the corpus luteum. *Proc. Natl. Acad. Sci.* **75**: 847.

Greenburg, G. and T. Hunt. 1978. The proliferative response in vitro of vascular endothelial and smooth muscle cells exposed to wound fluids and macrophages. *J. Cell. Physiol.* **97**: 353.

153

Hammarsten, J., A.C. Bylund-Fellenius, J. Holm, T. Schersten, and M. Krotkicwski. 1980. Capillary supply and muscle fibre types in patients with intermittent claudication: Relationships between morphology and metabolism. *Eur. J. Clin. Invest.* **10**: 301.

Hudlicka, O., R. Myrhage, and J. Cooper. 1977. Growth of capillaries in adult skeletal muscle after chronic stimulation. *Bibl. Anat.* **15**: 508.

Hunt, T., W. Andrews, B. Halliday, G. Greenburg, D. Knighton, R. Clark, and K. Thakral. 1981. Coagulation and macrophage stimulation of angiogenesis and wound healing. In *The surgical wound* (ed. P. Dineen and G. Hildick-Smith), p. 1. Lea and Febiger, Philadelphia.

Jakob, W., K.D. Jentzsh, D. Mauersberger, and P. Oehme. 1977. Demonstration of angiogenesis-activity in the corpus luteum of cattle. *Exp. Pathol.* **13**: 231.

Knighton, D., I. Silver, and T. Hunt. 1981. Regulation of wound-healing angiogenesis—Effect of oxygen gradients and inspired oxygen concentration. *Surgery* **90**: 262.

Knighton, D., T. Hunt, H. Scheuenstuhl, B. Halliday, Z. Werb, and M. Banda. 1983. Oxygen tension regulates the expression of angiogenesis factor by macrophages. *Science* **221**: 1283.

Makitie, H. 1977. Ultrastructure and density of skeletal muscle capillaries in atherosclerosis obliterans. *Bibl. Anat.* **16**: 380.

Polverini, P., R. Cotran, M. Gimbrone, and E. Unanue. 1977. Activated macrophages induce vascular proliferation. *Nature* **269**: 804.

Thakral, K., W. Goodson, and T. Hunt. 1979. Stimulation of wound blood vessel growth by wound macrophages. *J. Surg. Res.* **26**: 430.

Valdivia, E. 1958. Total capillary bed in striated muscle of guinea pigs native to the Peruvian mountains. *Am. J. Physiol.* **194**: 585.

154

Angiogenesis Induced by Normal Human Breast Tissue

H.M. Jensen

Department of Pathology, School of Medicine
University of California, Davis, California 95616

The ability to evoke a host response of new formation of capillaries (angiogenesis) is a common property of solid malignant neoplasms (Merwin and Algire 1956; Folkman 1971). The development of malignant tumors is believed to be a multistep process (Foulds 1954) and may take decades to evolve from initiation to the invasive step. The rabbit iris assay for angiogenesis factor (Gimbrone et al. 1973) has made it possible to ascertain at which step in malignant transformation angiogenesis factor is produced at increased levels.

Normal Human Breast

The mature female breast contains a branching duct tree on which the hormone-sensitive, potentially milk-producing microorgans, called lobules, are located peripherally. Thousands of 1–2-mm lobules are present in a breast, and each lobule is connected to the duct tree via a slender terminal duct. A lobule is composed of dozens of narrow, blindly ending test-tube-like glands called ductules. The structure of each lobule can be likened to a daisy with slender, delicate petals. Normally, the lobules atrophy in the perimenopausal years.

Site of Origin of Breast Cancer

In 2-mm-thick breast slices, the microarchitecture of breast parenchyma is displayed in three dimensions. Ductal carcinoma in situ originates in the terminal ductal lobular unit (Wellings and Jensen 1973); however, the ductules are few and coarse, but still connected by a slender terminal duct to the duct trees. The lesion can be likened to a tulip, in contrast to a daisy.

Cancer-associated breasts contain many cellular lesions that form a histologic continuum between normal lobules and ductal carcinoma in situ (Wellings et al. 1975). Statistical analyses indicated that these lesions are precancerous (Jensen et al. 1976). A retrospective study of thousands of biopsies showed that such lesions are associated with increased risk of later breast cancer (Dupont and Page 1985).

155

Table 1 Comparison of the Angiogenicity of Histologically Normal Lobules from Cancer Patients and Noncancer Patients

Days after transplantation	Angiogenicity[a]		
	cancer patients	noncancer patients	probability[b]
3	32/155 (21%)	21/307 (7%)	$p < 0.0001$ $\chi^2 = 17.992$
5	44/155 (28%)	46/307 (15%)	$p < 0.001$ $\chi^2 = 10.958$

[a]Number of lobules eliciting angiogenesis/total number assayed.
[b]Probability determined by Yate's corrected chi-square (χ^2).

Angiogenic Potential of Precancerous Lesions

Hyperplastic alveolar nodules, the precancerous lesions in the murine mammary gland, were found to be angiogenic on the rabbit iris (Gimbrone and Gullino 1976). The cellular human lesions, isolated after supravital staining with methylene blue chloride and deemed precancerous by histologic criteria, evoked angiogenesis in 30% of the cases, as did the murine precancerous lesions (Brem et al. 1978). Histologically normal-appearing lobules derived from cancer-associated breasts elicited angiogenesis in 28% of cases, whereas only 15% of such lobules obtained from benign biopsies did so. The data were similar regardless of the size of the lobule or the pre- versus postmenopausal status (Jensen et al. 1982) (Tables 1 and 2).

Table 2 Comparison of the Effects of Patient Age and Lobule Size on the Angiogenicity of Histologically Normal Lobules from Cancer Patients and Noncancer Patients

Attribute compared	Angiogenicity[a]	
	cancer patients	noncancer patients
Age of patients		
before 50 years	26/95 (27%)	43/279 (15%)
after 50 years	18/60 (30%) NS[b]	3/28 (10%) NS
Size of lobules		
<1 mm	30/112 (26%)	33/224 (14%)
>1 mm	14/43 (32%) NS	13/83 (15%) NS

[a]Number of lobules eliciting angiogenesis/total number assayed.
[b]NS = difference not statistically significant ($p > 0.05$) as determined by Yate's corrected chi-square.

DISCUSSION

These findings suggest that (1) the increased production of angiogenesis factor is a biologic marker for precancer; (2) the human breast at risk for cancer is diffusely afflicted, since 25–30% of its 5000–10,000 lobules are angiogenic; and (3) this change occurs before any histologic abnormalities are noted. It is a curious fact that women developing breast cancer retain the youthful succulent lobular parenchyma up to age 60, whereas in normal breasts, the lobules atrophy before age 50. Are the cancer-associated lobules retained because they produce more angiogenesis factor? Do they survive because of increased content of estrogen receptors or increased hormone stimulation? The abundance of the precancerous lobules makes it possible to study these tissues in which the origins of malignancy are likely to be found.

REFERENCES

Brem, S.S., H.M. Jensen, and P.M. Gullino. 1978. Angiogenesis as a marker of preneoplastic lesions of the human breast. *Cancer* **41**: 239.

Dupont, W.D. and D.L. Page. 1985. Risk factors for breast cancer in women with proliferative breast disease. *N. Engl. J. Med.* **312**: 146.

Folkman, J. 1971. Tumor angiogenesis: Therapeutic implications. *N. Engl. J. Med.* **285**: 1182.

Foulds, L. 1954. The experimental study of tumor progression: A review. *Cancer Res.* **14**: 327.

Gimbrone, M.A. and P.M. Gullino. 1976. Angiogenic capacity of preneoplastic lesions of the murine mammary gland as a marker of neoplastic transformation. *Cancer Res.* **36**: 2611.

Gimbrone, M.A., S.B. Leapman, R.S. Cotran, and J. Folkman. 1973. Tumor angiogenesis: Iris neovascularization at a distance from experimental intraocular tumors. *J. Natl. Cancer Inst.* **50**: 219.

Jensen, H.M., J.R. Rice, and S.R. Wellings. 1976. Preneoplastic lesions in the human breast. *Science* **191**: 295.

Jensen, H.M., I. Chen, M.R. DeVault, and A.E. Lewis. 1982. Angiogenesis induced by "normal" human breast tissue: A probable marker for precancer. *Science* **218**: 293.

Merwin, R.M. and G.H. Algire. 1956. The role of graft and host vessels in the vascularization of normal and neoplastic tissue. *J. Natl. Cancer Inst.* **17**: 23.

Wellings, S.R. and H.M. Jensen. 1973. On the origin and progression of ductal carcinoma of the human breast. *J. Natl. Cancer Inst.* **50**: 111.

Wellings, S.R., H.M. Jensen, and R.G. Marcum. 1975. An atlas of subgross pathology of the human breast with special reference to possible precancerous lesions. *J. Natl. Cancer Inst.* **55**: 231.

Closing Remarks

J. Folkman

Department of Surgery, Children's Hospital and Department of Surgery,
Anatomy, and Cellular Biology, Boston, Massachusetts 02115

Michael Klagsbrun and Daniel Rifkin asked me to make a few closing remarks. Some of you suggested that I give a brief history of this field, followed by a forecast; however, this does not seem to be an appropriate place to explore the beginnings of the field of angiogenesis or to try to predict its future direction. Anyone who has sat on a study section or has been the beneficiary of its deliberation must realize that there are no experts of the future, only experts of the past. Other participants at the meeting requested that the concluding session be used in order to come to agreement on a single name for the heparin-binding angiogenic factors related to fibroblast growth factor. I prefer, however, to leave this emotional issue of renaming factors to an institution like the World Health Organization.

Two aspects of the meeting stand out: (1) The superb reports by the molecular biologists have brought home to all of us the rapid progress that they have made during the past 2 years in refining angiogenic factors into distinct molecules. The consolation for those of us who work mainly in the slower discipline of cell biology must be that at least we have made the world of blood vessels safe for molecular biologists. (2) A free exchange of ideas between university and industrial scientists was successfully arranged by the organizers. A similar exchange probably would not have been possible a decade ago anywhere in this country. The success of the discussion periods was in no small part aided by the fact that FGF seems to be chemotactic to companies.

Several interesting questions have been raised for future consideration. For example, we have begun to use the term "direct" for angiogenic factors that stimulate capillary endothelial cell proliferation or locomotion in vitro and the term "indirect" for factors that do not. The indirect factors presumably mobilize macrophages to secrete their own direct angiogenic factor or utilize some other unknown mechanism. Is this distinction between direct and indirect angiogenic factors useful? Does it really matter that we try to identify the target of a given angiogenic factor? This distinction may be valid, especially for a patient with a nonhealing wound or fracture. One would want to treat such a patient with an angiogenic factor that could act independently of the cells whose deficiency may have been responsible for the delayed healing.

A more serious dilemma is that the definition of a direct angiogenic factor depends entirely on an in vitro bioassay. When endothelial cells proliferate or migrate in vivo in response to an angiogenic factor, one cannot be certain that the factor itself was the proximate cause of the endothelial cell stimulation. There is also the intriguing possibility that a factor may initiate angiogenesis indirectly but inhibit it directly. For example, Roberts and Sporn reported that TGF-β inhibits capillary endothelial cell proliferation in vitro but stimulates angiogenesis in vivo, presumably because it is strongly chemotactic for macrophages. This apparent paradox may be explained by the possibility that the macrophage chemotactic activity of TGF-β accounts for its initial angiogenic activity. As the release of angiogenic factor(s) from macrophages subsides, the endothelial cell inhibiting activity of TGF-β can be unmasked.

Another important question that has emerged is whether these well-characterized endothelial growth factors will eventually enlarge our understanding of the diseases dominated by abnormal angiogenesis, or possibly be employed to treat these diseases. After more than a decade of study of angiogenesis, a group of pathologic states are now being recognized as "angiogenic diseases," although they were previously thought to be unrelated. These diseases are managed by physicians in several specialties. They can be considered according to whether they can be ameliorated by either inhibition or stimulation of angiogenesis.

Patients who could benefit from treatment with an angiogenesis inhibitor include those with some of the following diseases: diabetic retinopathy, retrolental fibroplasia, corneal graft neovascularization, neovascular glaucoma, trachoma, psoriasis, pyogenic granuloma, hemangiomas, neovascularization in hemophiliac joints, angiofibromas, vascular adhesions, certain hypertrophic scars, and arthritis. The list should of course include solid tumors that are dependent on angiogenesis for progressive growth and metastasis. There are so many different kinds of pathologic ocular neovascularization that the development of a potent angiogenesis inhibitor could conceivably revolutionize ophthalmology. It is too early to predict whether such an inhibitor would act by specifically blocking an angiogenic factor or by suppressing capillary growth regardless of the mode of stimulation.

There are other pathologic states in which angiogenesis may be deficient and in which the administration of an angiogenic factor may be helpful. Examples of such abnormalities include the various types of delayed wound healing reported to us by Knighton et al. (this volume), scleroderma, and nonunion fractures. It is possible to consider the

160

enhancement of normal wound healing by angiogenic stimulators, as in burns and perhaps myocardial infarction.

The exciting reports in this volume have stimulated several new ideas about possible future directions for the study of angiogenesis. For example, we can ask: (1) What is the mechanism of low-molecular-weight angiogenic factors such as prostaglandins? Could some of them act by releasing angiogenic peptides from cells or extracellular matrix? (2) Does estrogen regulate any of the angiogenic factors discussed in this volume, e.g., ECGF, FGF, TGF-α, and TGF-β? There is still no biochemical link between female hormones and the neovascularization associated with ovulation, menstrual repair of the uterus, or development of the placenta. (3) Could a more efficient bioassay be developed for angiogenesis activity to substitute for the chick embryo chorioallantoic membrane or the rabbit cornea? (4) Is wound contracture dependent on neovascularization? (5) What is the role of mast cells in angiogenesis? (6) How is lumen formation initiated in a growing capillary sprout? Is it dependent on any of the known growth factors? These questions and many more indicate that much experimental work remains to be done before we reach an understanding of angiogenesis that is as sophisticated as our picture of phenomena such as blood coagulation.

161